Barbara Rief Vernay, Iris Mach (Eds.)

How Pandemics Shape the Metropolitan Space

How Pandemics Shape the Metropolitan Space

Impact of COVID-19
on Urban Development in Vienna and Tokyo

edited by

Barbara Rief Vernay and Iris Mach

LIT

Cover images:
Empty Shibuya Station, Tokyo (Photo: Takeru Shibayama)
Empty Karlsplatz Station, Vienna (Photo: Takeru Shibayama)

Gefördert von der Stadt Wien Kultur und JASEC, TU Wien
Funded by Stadt Wien Kultur and JASEC, TU Wien

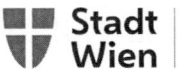 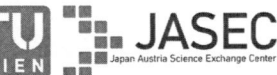

English proofreading:
Robert D. E. Senior, Vienna
Gabriele Berghammer, Vienna

Bibliographic information published by the Deutsche Nationalbibliothek
The Deutsche Nationalbibliothek lists this publication in the Deutsche Nationalbibliografie; detailed bibliographic data are available on the Internet at http://dnb.dnb.de.

ISBN 978-3-643-91238-1 (pb)
ISBN 978-3-643-96238-6 (PDF)

A catalogue record for this book is available from the British Library.

© LIT VERLAG GmbH & Co. KG Wien 2023
Contact:
Garnisongasse 1/19
A-1090 Wien
Tel. +43 (0) 1-409 56 61   Fax +43 (0) 1-409 56 97
E-Mail: wien@lit-verlag.at   https://www.lit-verlag.at
Distribution:
In the UK: Global Book Marketing, e-mail: mo@centralbooks.com

Contents

Preface 7
Iris Mach

Introduction 9
Barbara Rief Vernay, Iris Mach

CHAPTER 1: New Housing Preferences as a Result of the Pandemic

The Pandemic as a Driver of Urban Flight?
A Study on the Vienna Metropolitan Area 23
Barbara Rief Vernay, Iris Mach

Polarised Residential Preferences for the Centre and
Outer Suburban Tokyo After the Experience of COVID-19 41
*Keisuke Sakamoto, Takahiro Yamazaki, Toru Terada, Noriko Akita,
Akito Murayama, Akiko Iida, Marco Amati, Makoto Yokohari*

CHAPTER 2: The Transformation of Public Space

The Streets of Vienna in Times of the COVID-19
Pandemic - Transformation Processes of Public Space Through
Walking, Cycling and Scootering 77
Irene Bittner

Impact of the COVID-19 Pandemic on Public Space in Tokyo 91
Rinpei Miura

CHAPTER 3: Public Transport Amid and After the Crisis

Public Transport in Vienna and Tokyo Amid and
After the COVID-19 Pandemic   115
Takeru Shibayama

CHAPTER 4: Pandemic and Urban Culture

Displaced Youth and Culture:
Informal Art and Culture During the COVID-19 Measures
in Vienna and Future Potentials for Public Space   141
Fabian Dembski

Culture and COVID-19: Tokyo's Classical Music Concert Halls on
Their Way Back to Being Monofunctional Spaces   157
Masayasu Komiya

CHAPTER 5: Urban Green Space and Health Crises

Vienna's Urban Green Space as an Element of Resilience
in Times of Epidemics   177
Meinhard Breiling

Urban Green Space Planning for New Work Styles
in the Post-Pandemic Era   199
*Takahiro Yamazaki, Akiko Iida, Kimihiro Hino, Akito Murayama,
U Hiroi, Toru Terada, Hideki Koizumi, Makoto Yokohari*

The Contributors   229

Preface

As a result of the global COVID-19 pandemic, cities around the world faced challenges that were unprecedented in their scale and scope. Large urban areas were particularly burdened due to complex functional interdependencies, but also because of high population densities that entailed an increased probability of infection. Three years after it began, it has become clear that the pandemic has reorganised urban space in both the short and the long term.

This volume examines the impact of the COVID-19 crisis on the metropolitan development of Vienna and Tokyo. Comparing two cities like these is a risky undertaking given their dissimilarities. The central European metropolis of Vienna differs from the Japanese metropolis of Tokyo not only in terms of population and area – equally incomparable are the historical and cultural conditions that have produced the respective building and administrative structures. However, with the COVID-19 pandemic, these vastly different cities faced the same global challenge. The question arises as to how each city has dealt with this crisis and to what extent cultural framework conditions influence solutions and strategies.

In June 2021, the Japan Austria Science Exchange Center (JASEC), Vienna University of Technology, together with the Graduate School of Frontier Sciences, University of Tokyo held a seminar titled "Vienna – Tokyo: Impact of COVID-19 on Urban Development". The aim was to approach the question from an interdisciplinary perspective, which was achieved through contributions from areas such as urban geography, regional planning but also landscape planning. The seminar lectures offered an original cross-sectional analysis and revealed not only differences but also commonalities in dealing with the crisis.

Thanks to a grant from the Department of Arts and Culture of the City of Vienna (MA 7), the valuable support of LIT Academic Publishing and the collaboration of the University of Tokyo, the Japan Austria Science Exchange Center was able to gather the contents of the conference in a modified and updated form in the present volume. In addition to the seminar papers, further relevant articles from the fields of transportation planning, urban sociology and cultural anthropology were included.

The Vienna University of Technology has maintained a cooperation with the University of Tokyo since 1981. Besides promoting the mobility of researchers and students, JASEC also supports scientific exchange on current topics in architectural and urban research. Crisis and disaster management is one of the institute's research foci; the topic "COVID-19 crisis and urban development" falls within this field.

Iris Mach
Head of JASEC (Vienna University of Technology), spring 2023

Introduction

Barbara Rief Vernay, Iris Mach

The outbreak of the SARS-CoV-2 pandemic led to a global health crisis in the early 2020s that is slowly subsiding after a duration of three years. Governments and local authorities have found themselves forced to apply regulatory policies to contain the spread of the virus and its variants. While drugs and vaccinations to counter the virus were still being developed, lockdowns were imposed along with other restrictions. These emergency measures, which were implemented more or less strictly depending on the country or region, affected everyday life at different levels.

At the macro level, there were temporary disruptions in global economic cycles and supply chain failures.[1] Tourism came to an almost complete standstill throughout the world.

But also at the local level, especially in urban areas, the pandemic led to major disturbances. In many places, public transport was severely restricted, non-essential shops, leisure and cultural facilities were forced to close, people were obliged to work from home wherever possible and education at all levels had to take place via distance learning (i.e. virtually). The main argument for this was to safeguard critical infrastructures[2], especially health facilities, which had to cope with a sudden and massive increase in the number of sick people.[3]

Urban areas and large cities in particular face special challenges in crisis situations such as the COVID pandemic. They have both high-density housing and high population density. They are also characterised by a strong interconnection

---

[1] Farrer, "Shanghai's 'grim' Covid outbreak threatens more global supply chain disruption."
[2] Critical infrastructures are facilities, systems that are essential for the maintenance of essential societal functions (health, safety, communication, economy, social well-being of the population, see also Document 32008L0114, European Council Directive 2008/114/EC)
[3] Lusa, "Health system on brink of collapse as COVID-19 cases surge."

of functions[4] being administrative centres and international transport hubs, controlling extensive local transport networks and serving as commuter centres for suburban areas. As higher-level centres, they also have supra-regional or global functions such as linking regional, national and international flows of finance, services and goods.[5] The vulnerability of large cities is thus due to a higher risk of contagion, but also to the fact that crisis-related disruptions of urban systems have particularly severe effects there, even beyond the city itself.

On the other hand, large urban spaces are places of innovation and creativity. Large cities have resources that enable them to develop original strategies for coping with crises. Globally established strategies such as *Smart City* or *Urban Resilience* are examples of cities' efforts to find innovative solutions. The former are intended to make cities more sustainable through technical, economic and social innovations[6], the latter aim at counteracting threatening events caused by nature and humans (e. g., climate change, migration, economic crises, etc.) in a preventative manner, while at the same time compensating for the consequences of crises. Resilience, the ability of a system to return to a previously stable state after stressful events[7], is of particular importance for cities in the COVID and post-COVID context.

Epidemics as a driver of urban transformation

Crisis management in the context of epidemics, however, is not a new experience for cities. During the last centuries, infectious diseases have repeatedly disrupted cities and ultimately caused long-term spatial changes. Sakamoto et al. mention in this volume that the phenomena of urban flight and suburbanisation have existed in cities like London since the 17th century and were mainly triggered by successive waves of infectious diseases.

On the other hand, epidemics led to the creation of new health-promoting urban development concepts. In fact, between the Enlightenment and the late 19th century, disease control and hygiene efforts were the main drivers of urban modernisation.

However, the argument of disease control and the related urban planning was also used by local authorities to control the population, as Michel Foucault

---

[4] Matheson et al., "Why has coronavirus affected cities more than rural areas?"
[5] Sassen, "Cities and Communities in the Global Economy: Rethinking Our Concepts."
[6] SmartCitiesWorld.
[7] Resilience is the ability of a system to return to a previous stable state following stressors caused by any hazard. (see also McGill, "Urban resilience – an Urban Management Perspective.").

points out in the chapter *"Le panoptisme"* of his work *"Surveiller et punir. Naissance de la prison"* (Discipline and Punish: The Birth of the Prison). Foucault describes the implementation of strict policing measures to contain a plague epidemic in late 17th century Paris. According to the author, authorities instrumentalised the public health argument to justify increased regulation and surveillance of urban life to move closer to the "utopia of the perfectly governed city"[8].

The smallpox epidemics of 18th century Paris were contained without resort to such draconian measures, i.e. through empirical measurements, through scientific observation (later also through vaccination), but above all through improved urban conditions. The urban planning ideals of the Enlightenment were thus not only driven by representative motives, but also by a sustained concern for hygiene. For example, Pierre Charles L'Enfant's 1791 urban design for Washington, D.C. was inspired by then new medical discoveries such as that of the circulation of blood. L'Enfant sought to create a healthy environment through highly organised urban planning – wide boulevards and straight, interconnected streets were to make the city a "healthy body" with a "clean skin" in which movement could take place and breath could circulate.[9]

With advancing industrialisation in the 19th century, urban growth and the associated air pollution, along with newly emerging epidemics such as cholera, considerations of hygiene became even more important for urban planning. Cholera broke out several times in Vienna between 1836 and 1873, in Tokyo (formerly 'Edo') in the 1820s, in 1858 and in 1862. Paris was badly affected in 1832. With the slogan *"Paris embellie, Paris agrandie, Paris assainie"* (expand, embellish and clean up Paris), French official Baron Haussmann emphasised the importance of containing epidemics in connection with the Paris urban redevelopment program carried out from 1850. The redevelopment projects of Barcelona, Berlin, Vienna, and Budapest were also guided by the principles of 19th century hygienism[10]. This not only included the construction of wide, straight streets with plain paving, but also the installation of sewage systems, the supply of clean water and the construction of large, highly specialised health facilities.

Planners of non-European cities also applied strategies to prevent epidemics and other diseases. For example, New York's Central Park, completed by Frederic Law Olmsted in 1873 on the European model, was inspired by the

---

[8] Foucault, *Surveiller et punir. Naissance de la prison*, 200.
[9] Sennett, *Flesh and Stone. The Body and the City in Western Civilization*, 263.
[10] Le Roux, "Le siècle des hygiénistes."

need to create healthy recreational spaces within the city.[11] The concept for the modernisation of Tokyo drawn up by the physician and politician Goto Shimpei in 1890 was also based on hygiene-related considerations.[12]

Health, air, light and clarity were also key elements of modernist urban planning in the 20th century. From the end of the 19th century, cities had grown rapidly. Resulting problems such as dilapidated buildings and poor housing conditions had already led to a paradigm shift in urban planning at the beginning of the 20th century. Instead of conventional dense block perimeter layouts, planners propagated open layouts with extensive green spaces. Under the chairmanship of the French architect Le Corbusier, the association CIAM (*Congrès International d'Architecture Moderne,* 1928–1959) formulated new principles for the urban development of the future[13] – large-scale planning on a tabula rasa was to put an end to the chaos of the 19th century city. According to CIAM, it was no longer the people but the city itself that was "sick". In his work *"Manière de penser l'urbanisme. Soigner la ville malade"* (A way of conceiving urbanism. Healing the sick city)[14] Le Corbusier described how modern technology and functional separation could be used to "cure" the "sick city [of the 19th century]". The model of the *Functional City* (prefabricated housing estates on the outskirts of towns and new satellite towns) that emerged from this movement, however, was realised only in the post-war decades in many parts of the world.

Urban density and crisis

From the 1970s onwards, growing criticism of the modernist *Functional City* led to a return to the qualities of the hitherto neglected inner-city spaces.[15] Due to the common practice of vaccination against lethal infectious diseases from the middle of the 20th century, the threat of epidemics no longer existed and urban authorities concentrated their resources on other issues, such as the renewal of historic cores. Comprehensive redevelopment policies brought the upper middle class of Europe, America and Asia back to central, densely built-up areas within a few decades.[16] Thus, the paradigm of the *Functional city* was replaced by that of the *Compact city*. The latter, still valid today, is characterised by high residential

---

[11] Beveridge, *Mount Royal in the works of Frederick Law Olmsted,* 43.
[12] Sorensen, *The Making of Urban Japan. Cities and Planning from Edo to the Twenty First Century,* 87.
[13] Mumford, *The CIAM Discourse on Urbanism 1928- 1960.*
[14] Le Corbusier, *Manière de penser l'urbanisme. Soigner la ville malade.*
[15] Bidou-Zachariasen, *Retours en ville.*
[16] Plater-Zyberk, "The Charter of the New Urbanism."

densities and mixed land use, and is intended to promote a high density of interaction in the public space, as well as pedestrian and bicycle traffic.

With the onset of the pandemic and the lockdowns that followed, the idea of the *Compact city* was put to the test. Unable to leave their homes, city dwellers experienced compactness and density in a new way. The lack of green space, the lack of open space generally, and the fact that urban housing tends to be smaller than rural housing sparked discussions about the legitimacy of building densities in cities. However, the pandemic has shown that in crisis situations with supply and logistical problems, the most resilient urban areas are precisely those where facilities for daily supplies and other important infrastructure can be found within walking or cycling distance. In this context, the *15-minute-city* conceived by Colombian urbanist Carlos Moreno has gained new attention. In 2016, Moreno had already reconceptualised the idea of walkability, which had been postulated since the 1980s, as the *15-minute city*. It provides urban dwellers with six essential functions within a 15-minute walk or bike ride: housing, work, commerce, health, education and entertainment.[17] The *15-minute city* differs from the *Compact city* in that it also takes into account issues such as climate change, new technologies, the sharing economy, and cultural and social needs.[18]

The metropolitan regions of Vienna and Tokyo, which are the subject of this volume, are both based on the concept of the compact city. Vienna's urban planning is based entirely on this concept,[19] while Tokyo has not adopted it across the board due to decentralised administrative structures. Both cities report having positive experiences during the pandemic with "high quality density"[20] that has a functional mix to serve a variety of needs[21].

Vienna and Tokyo: A European metropolis and an Asian megacity

According to the Global Cities Index (Kearney), Tokyo ranked fourth worldwide in 2022, and Vienna 20th[22]. With a population of over 37 million, the

---

[17] Moreno et al., "Introducing the '15-Minute City': Sustainability, Resilience and Place Identity in Future Post-Pandemic Cities," 100.
[18] Ibid., 101.
[19] Stadt Wien, Magistratsabteilung 18 "Stadtentwicklung und Stadtplanung", "STEP 2025. Stadtentwicklungsplan Wien," 49.
[20] Häberlin et al., "Corona: Die Rolle der Stadtplanung für die Krisenbewältigung am Beispiel Wien."
[21] Shimizu, Murooka and Taniguchi, "Realizing a 15-minute city in Metropolitan Tokyo."
[22] Kearney, "2022 Global Cities Report."

Greater Tokyo area is classified as a megacity, while the Vienna metropolitan area with 2.9 million inhabitants corresponds to a typical Central European metropolitan area. There are differing opinions on where one should delimit the metropolitan areas of Vienna and Tokyo, which makes a direct comparison difficult. The Vienna *Stadtregion Plus*[23] has 2.9 million inhabitants (2019)[24] in an area of 7,595 km2 (a total of 269 municipalities being the city of Vienna plus 205 municipalities in the federal state of Lower Austria and 63 municipalities in the federal state of Burgenland). With 37.2 million inhabitants[25], *Greater Tokyo Area* is the largest built-up area in the world[26], covering 13,500 km2 and consisting of the metropolis of Tokyo and the prefectures of Chiba, Gunma, Ibaraki, Kanagawa, Saitama, Tochigi and Yamanashi.

As far as the municipal areas of Vienna and Tokyo are concerned, the delimitation is clearer. Vienna is defined by its administrative boundaries; the city is divided into 23 districts, covers 415 km2 and has 1.93 million inhabitants.[27] In the case of Tokyo, one must distinguish between the Tokyo prefecture area and the central city area. The prefecture comprises the central city area and another 30 municipalities.[28] The central city area covers 621 km2 and has 9.64 million inhabitants.[29] Like Vienna, it is divided in 23 administrative units (Wards).[30]

The current built structures of the two cities have come about due to very different growth processes: Vienna's structure is, as is typical for European cities, the result of centuries of concentric growth. Vienna's city centre is the geographical centre and the place of its first settlement. To this day it is the

---

[23] We refer to the delimitation defined by the spatial planning group Planungsgemeinschaft Ost (POG). This delimitation has no administrative relevance, it is an artificial line which has been drawn for spatial planning issues. (see also Rief Vernay and Mach in this volume).

[24] Ringler et al., „Wohnen und Leben in der Stadtregion+: Endbericht zur Studie," 15.

[25] "Demographia World Urban Areas (Built up Urban Areas or World Agglomerations), 18th Annual Edition," 21.

[26] "Statistical Handbook of Japan."

[27] As of January 2022 (Statistics Austria).

[28] The number rises to 39 if one includes a town and eight villages on the far-flung islands south of Tokyo (Izu and Ogasawara Islands), which are administratively part of Tokyo Prefecture but are not normally counted as part of the Tokyo metropolitan area.

[29] As of March 2021 (e-Stat).

[30] Like Vienna, today's Tokyo metropolitan area was formed by the merger of formerly independent municipalities. While the administrative incorporation of Viennese suburbs such as Währing, Ottakring and Hütteldorf took place as early as 1892 (in the course of late 19th century urban renewal), cities such as Shibuya, Shinjuku and Ikebukuro were not incorporated into Tokyo's urban area until 1932. However, while the districts in Vienna do not have far-reaching decision-making powers, the wards in Tokyo are autonomous units with elected mayors. The wards can, for example, define their own urban development concepts.

focus of political, cultural and also economic life. The inner-city area is characterised by a largely well-preserved late 19th century block perimeter development. The adjacent urban expansion areas built from the second half of the 20th century onwards are mostly marked by open layout structures (e.g. large scale housing estates)[31].

Tokyo's built structure does not conform to concentric growth logic. It shows locally very different morphological features and is based less on large-scale global urban planning than on a complex interplay of legal, economic and administrative conditions[32]. Unlike Vienna or other European cities, Tokyo does not have one city centre that is also the historical centre and the centre of all urban functions. In his work on the semiotics of the city, the French theorist Roland Barthes noted in the early 1970s that Tokyo did have a kind of centre, but that this centre was entirely occupied by the imperial palace, itself surrounded by a deep moat and hidden in the green. The centre of Tokyo (formerly Edo Castle) was thus "not the culmination of any particular activity" but a kind of "void necessary for the organisation of the rest of the city"[33]. If one considers multifunctional urban reference points as city centres, in Tokyo, the areas around the major railway stations, where the terminus of the busy private railway lines are connected to the ring railway (Yamanote Line), are such centres. The multitude of these form a polycentric structure. In Vienna, too, numerous sub-centres form a polycentric structure, but functionally and culturally the Viennese sub-centres clearly rank below the main centre.

Since the beginning of the 20th century, Vienna has experienced profound urban innovations, mainly through the urbanisation and transformation of its peripheral areas. Tokyo has also undergone several large-scale renewals during the same time period, especially after the great Kanto earthquake of 1923, after the air raids on Tokyo in 1945, and finally with the hosting of the 1964 Olympic Games. Since the mid-1990s, Tokyo has also been transforming itself from a city of predominantly low buildings into a "city of towers"[34].

Metropolises reshaped by the pandemic

Both metropolitan areas face individual challenges. Tokyo has to be prepared for seismic events at any time, the city also has to deal with the problem of an aging population, while Vienna has to cope with a dramatic population

---

[31] Tamáska, *Metropolen. Parallele Stadträume aus dem 20. Jahrhundert*, 32–47.
[32] Perez, "The Historical Development of the Tokyo Skyline: Timeline and Morphology," 609.
[33] Barthes, "Sémiologie et Urbanisme," 12.
[34] Perez, "The Historical Development of the Tokyo Skyline: Timeline and Morphology," 609.

increase due to immigration. There are also global urban challenges that are relevant to both metropolitan areas, albeit on different scales – increasing interurban competitive pressure, climate change, growing pollution, a lack of affordable housing, growing socio-spatial disparities and urban sprawl. Add to this the COVID-19 crisis and the possibility of further pandemics in the future.[35] Managing urban transformation triggered by the global health crisis and developing long-term resilience is a new challenge.

The approach to urban challenges and crises taken by the two cities differs greatly. Firstly because of their scales – "urban exodus" tendencies, for example, have unequal effects in a megapolis with 37 million inhabitants and a Central European metropolitan area with barely three million inhabitants. Secondly, local cultural conditions and the historical paths taken by their institutions have proven decisive in determining how they act in a crisis: Vienna's highly centralised city government, which has existed for over 100 years, operates differently from one of the 23 independent district councils within Tokyo's likewise historically anchored system of local government. Also, the use of public spaces during lockdown had a different dynamic in a European city with a strong culture of civil society than in a Japanese city where civil society participation in urban policy issues is only just emerging.

This volume examines the impact of the recent pandemic crisis on the urban development of the Vienna and Tokyo metropolitan areas. It aims to make clear that the COVID-19 pandemic, just like epidemics of past centuries, reshapes cities not only in the short term but also in the long term.

The volume is divided into five chapters. It covers the topics of internal migration, public space, public transport, urban culture and urban green spaces.

In the first chapter, Barbara Rief Vernay, Iris Mach, Keisuke Sakamoto, Takahiro Yamazaki, Toru Terada, Noriko Akita, Akito Murayama, Akiko Iida, Marco Amati and Makoto Yokohari focus on the question of whether COVID-19 has led to new housing preferences within the respective metropolitan area in the medium and long term. In the second chapter, Irene Bittner and Rinpei Miura show how civil society reclaimed public space in many places during the crisis but how elsewhere public space was transformed into commercial space. In the third chapter, Takeru Shibayama describes the situation of public transport in both cities before and after the start of the pandemic. In the fourth chapter, Fabian Dembski and Masayasu Komiya investigate changes in urban cultural life. Dembski focuses on new cultural practices of Viennese

---

[35] Park, "Why Infectious Disease Outbreaks Are Becoming So Common."

youth and young adults, while Komiya presents the impact of the pandemic on Tokyo institutions of high culture. In the fifth and last chapter, Meinhard Breiling, Takahiro Yamazaki, Akiko Iida, Kimihiro Hino, Akito Murayama, U Hiroi, Toru Terada, Hideki Koizumi and Makoto Yokohari examine how the COVID-19 crisis has changed the function and significance of urban green spaces.

Bibliography

"Demographia World Urban Areas (Built up Urban Areas or World Agglomerations), 18th Annual Edition." Accessed January 31, 2023. http://www.demographia.com/db-worldua.pdf.

"Statistical Handbook of Japan." Accessed January 31, 2023. https://www.stat.go.jp/english/data/handbook/c0117.htm#cha2_6.

Barthes, Roland. "Sémiologie Et Urbanisme." *L'Architecture d'aujourd'hui*, no. 53 (1970/1971): 11–13.

Beveridge, Charles E. *Mount Royal in the Works of Frederick Law Olmsted*. Montréal, 2002. Accessed November 12, 2022. https://www.mcgill.ca/urbanplanning/files/urbanplanning/mount_royal_in_the_works_of_frederick_law_olmsted.pdf.

Bidou-Zachariasen, Catherine. Daniel Hiernaux Nicolas, and Hélène Rivière d'Arc, eds. *Retours En Ville*. Collection "Les urbanites". Paris: Descartes, 2003.

e-Stat. https://www.e-stat.go.jp/.

Farrer, Martin. "Shanghai's 'Grim' Covid Outbreak Threatens More Global Supply Chain Disruption." *The Guardian*, April 6, 2022. Accessed November 2, 2022. https://www.theguardian.com/business/2022/apr/06/shanghais-grim-covid-outbreak-threatens-more-global-supply-chain-disruption.

Foucault, Michel. *Surveiller Et Punir. Naissance De La Prison*. Paris: Gallimard, 1975.

Häberlin, Udo, Gerlinde Mückstein, Nils Peters, Gregor Stratil-Sauer, Johannes Suitner, Tobias Troger, and Maria Wasserburger. "Corona: Die Rolle Der Stadtplanung für Die Krisenbewältigung Am Beispiel Wien." In *REAL CORP 2020: Shaping Urban Change - Livable City Regions for the 21st Century: Proceedings of the 25th International Conference on Urban Planning, Regional Development and Information Society 15-18 September 2020, Virtual Conference = Beiträge zur 25. Internationalen Konferenz zu Stadtplanung, Regionalentwicklung und Informationsgesellschaft*. Edited by Manfred Schrenk et al. 2nd edition, 1271–81. Vienna: CORP – Competence Center of Urban and Regional Planning, 2020.

Jesse, Matheson, Max Nathan, Harry Pickard, and Enrico Vanino. "Why Has Coronavirus Affected Cities More Than Rural Areas?" *Economics Observatory*, July 2, 2020. Accessed November 3, 2022. https://www.economicsobservatory.com/why-has-coronavirus-affected-cities-more-rural-areas.

Kearney. "2022 Global Cities Report." Accessed January 31, 2023. https://www.kearney.com/industry/public-sector/global-cities/2022.

Le Corbusier. *Manière De Penser L'urbanisme. Soigner La Ville Malade.* Paris: Denoël/Gonthier, 1997.

Le Roux, Thomas. "Le Siècle Des Hygiénistes." *La Vie des idées*, 06/2010. Accessed November 12, 2022. https://laviedesidees.fr/Le-siecle-des-hygienistes.html.

Lusa. "Health System on Brink of Collapse as COVID-19 Cases Surge." January 18, 2021. Accessed November 2, 2022. https://www.theportugalnews.com/news/2021-01-18/health-system-on-brink-of-collapse-as-covid-19-cases-surge/57771.

McGill, Ronald. "Urban Resilience – an Urban Management Perspective." *Journal of Urban Management* 9, no. 3 (2020): 372–81.

Moreno, Carlos, Zaheer Allam, Didier Chabaud, Catherine Gall, and Florent Pratlong. "Introducing the '15-Minute City': Sustainability, Resilience and Place Identity in Future Post-Pandemic Cities." *Smart Cities* 4, no. 1 (2021): 93–111. https://doi.org/10.3390/smartcities4010006.

Mumford, Eric. *The CIAM Discourse on Urbanism 1928-1960.* Cambridge: the MIT Press, 2000.

Park, Alice. "Why Infectious Disease Outbreaks Are Becoming So Common." September 15, 2022. Accessed February 3, 2023. https://time.com/6211430/infectious-disease-outbreaks-polio-covid-19/.

Perez, Rafael Ivan Pazos. "The Historical Development of the Tokyo Skyline: Timeline and Morphology." *Journal of Asian Architecture and Building Engineering* 13, no. 3 (2014): 609–15. https://doi.org/10.3130/jaabe.13.609.

Plater-Zyberk, Elizabeth. "The Charter of the New Urbanism." Accessed January 31, 2023. https://www.cnu.org/sites/default/files/Plater-zyberk_charter.pdf.

Ringler, Paul, Bernhard Hoser, Ogris Günther, and David Laumer. "Wohnen und Leben in der Stadtregion+: Endbericht zur Studie." Accessed January 31, 2023. https://www.planungsgemeinschaft-ost.at/fileadmin/root_pgo/Studien/Raumordnung/Leben_und_Wohnen_in_der_Sadtregion__Analysebericht.pdf.

Sassen, Saskia. "Cities and Communities in the Global Economy: Rethinking Our Concepts." *American Behavioral Scientist* 39, no. 5 (1996): 629–39. https://doi.org/10.1177/0002764296039005009.

Sennett, Richard. *The Body and the City in Western Civilization.* New York: W. W. Norton & Company, 1994.

Shimizu, Hiroki, Taichi Murooka, and Mamoru Taniguchi. "Realizing a 15-Minute City in Metropolitan Tokyo." *Journal of the City Planning Institute of Japan* 57, no. 3 (2022): 592–98. https://doi.org/10.11361/journalcpij.57.592.

SmartCitiesWorld. Accessed November 20, 2022. https://www.smartcitiesworld.net/home.

Sorensen, André. *The Making of Urban Japan: Cities and Planning from Edo to the Twenty-First Century.* London: Routledge, 2004.

Stadt Wien, Magistratsabteilung 18 „Stadtentwicklung und Stadtplanung". "STEP 2025. Stadtentwicklungsplan Wien." Accessed January 31, 2023. https://www.wien.gv.at/stadtentwicklung/studien/pdf/b008379a.pdf.

Statistics Austria. Accessed January 31, 2023. https //www.statistik.at/en/statistics/population-and-society/population/population-stock/population-at-beginning-of-year/quarter.

Tamáska, Máté. *Metropolen Budapest Wien: Parallele Stadträume aus dem 20. Jahrhundert.* Architektur im Ringturm L. Salzburg: Müry Salzmann Verlag, 2018.

CHAPTER 1:

New Housing Preferences as a Result of the Pandemic

The Pandemic as a Driver of Urban Flight? A Study on the Vienna Metropolitan Area

Barbara Rief Vernay, Iris Mach

"Die digitalen Nomaden, die mit ihrem Laptop von überall auf der Welt arbeiten können, ziehen aufs Land oder in eine der sogenannten ‚Zoom towns', die neue Bewohner mit Prämien anlocken. Das Leben dort ist billiger, die Luft besser."[1]

As recently as 2018 and 2019, Vienna ranked first in the British Economist's "Global Livability Ranking". With the COVID-19 crisis of 2020, however, the "world's most livable city" appeared to have lost much of its appeal, dropping to 12th place in 2021.[2] It seems that the pandemic and the social distancing, lockdowns, and curfews imposed to curb the spread of the virus have exposed the deficits of major cities like Vienna. In densely built-up core areas, housing is usually expensive, apartments are small, and private outdoor and public green spaces are scarce. Restrictions on cultural life and the heavy strains a pandemic places on healthcare infrastructures further compounded these challenges.[3] At the same time, the advent of digitalisation has opened up new possibilities for living and working in virtual space, allowing people to leave the city and its disadvantages behind and escape to the rural-like suburban belt.

"Urban flight", therefore, has become a buzzword increasingly frequently seen in Austrian media reports since 2021. The focus is on Vienna and its suburban areas—which are expected to gain population due to urban flight. Yet, even long before the pandemic, the scattered urban growth sprawling to

---

[1] "The digital nomads, who can work from anywhere in the world with their laptops, are moving to the countryside or to one of the so-called 'zoom towns,'. Life there is cheaper, and the air better." (Lobe, "Ortlose Gesellschaft. Stadtflucht: Wer braucht noch Orte?").
[2] Fabry, „Corona kostet Wien den Titel ‚lebenswerteste Stadt'."
[3] "Wien verliert ‚Economist'-Titel als lebenswerteste Stadt."

suburban areas has been one of Austria's major environmental concerns, particularly against a backdrop of climate change and scarce resources.[4]

This article discusses the effects of the COVID-19 pandemic on migration movements between the core city of Vienna and its suburban areas. We will first introduce the Vienna metropolitan area, which covers the city of Vienna and suburban municipalities. We will then analyse the population trends in suburban municipalities to determine whether these have experienced a disproportionate population increase since the beginning of the pandemic and explore the evolution of demand for real estate and of real estate prices in these areas.

The Vienna metropolitan area

Depending on the purpose, there are a number of definitions of what constitutes the Vienna metropolitan area. We will here use the definition proposed by the planning association *Planungsgemeinschaft Ost* (PGO), a joint organisation of the federal provinces of Vienna, Lower Austria, and Burgenland, in 1978, as it best accommodates the functional relationships between the core city and suburban areas that are relevant for our analysis. The concept of a 'Vienna metropolitan area' has no administrative or historical-cultural significance; its demarcation merely serves to coordinate regional developmental activities between the federal provinces of Vienna, Lower Austria, and Burgenland in areas such as transport and mobility, economy, green spaces, energy, or climate protection.

The Vienna metropolitan area is located in the east of Austria and covers an area of 7,595 km2. Its outer border is a distance of 40 to 60 km from the city centre of Vienna. In the south and east, metropolitan Vienna is delimited by Hungarian and Slovakian national borders, in the north by the municipalities of Hollabrunn and Mistelbach, and in the west by the foothills of the Vienna Woods. The area includes the federal capital, Vienna, with its 23 districts as well as 205 municipalities in the federal province of Lower Austria and 63 municipalities in the federal province of Burgenland. The Vienna metropolitan area is the economically strongest region in Austria and, due to its well-developed infrastructures and excellent accessibility, among Europe's most dynamic urban regions.[5]

---

[4] Lindenthal and Schlatzer, *Risiken für die Lebensmittelversorgung in Österreich und Lösungsansätze für eine höhere Krisensicherheit, Diskussionspapier des Zentrums für globalen Wandel und Nachhaltigkeit*, 22.
[5] PGO (Planungsgemeinschaft Ost).

In terms of urban development, metropolitan Vienna can be divided into three concentric zones. At its heart is the 19th century core city, which is mainly located on the right bank of the river Danube. It is characterised by its block perimeter development and high-density construction. The core city is surrounded by a transition zone dominated in the west by the natural space of the Vienna Woods and in the northeast to southwest by inhomogeneous, mostly open-layout developments of post-war decades and recent settlements. The third and outermost zone is the suburban area outside the administrative city boundary of Vienna. It features a mix of former rural areas, extensive areas with single-family homes, and isolated structures, such as shopping malls and retail centres. The scattered spatial patterns in this zone are the result of suburbanisation processes that began in the 1950s and continue to this day (Fig. 1).

Urban flight and suburbanisation between the 1950s and the 2010s

In terms of size, built-up Vienna continued to correspond to its 19th century version well into the early 1950s. Expansion beyond the city's administrative boundaries did not start until the post-war economic upswing of the mid-1950s. The European Recovery Program (ERP), or "Marshall Plan", strengthened the industrial and tertiary sectors from 1953 onwards.[6] New large-scale industrial areas were first set up in the federal province of Lower Austria south of Vienna. Completion of the northern section of the southbound A2 motorway in 1962 was a prerequisite for the establishment of *Industriezentrum Niederösterreich Süd (IZ NÖ-Süd)*, the first business park of Lower Austria and still the largest of its kind in Austria.[7]

The 1962 *Planungskonzept Wien*,[8] a planning concept developed by architect and head of urban planning, Roland Rainer, provided a comprehensive regional planning framework for further expansion of the city. The concept was consistent with the then prevailing paradigm of the 'functional city,' which aimed at separating urban functions by land-use zoning and moving industry from the inner city to the periphery. Along this vein, the planning concept contained guidelines for establishing new development axes and a transportation system that anticipated the outward expansion of the city into the federal province of Lower Austria.[9] Satellite cities such as in France or the USA were not envisaged for Vienna. Rather, the large-scale public residential development program focused on prefabricated housing estates along the edges of the 19th century city.

---

[6] Platzer, "Wien, ein Sonderfall im ‚Kalten Krieg'?," 77.
[7] Hartl, "Wanderungsbewegungen an die Peripherie der Stadt Wien," 254.
[8] Rainer, *Planungskonzept Wien*.
[9] Ibid., 87.

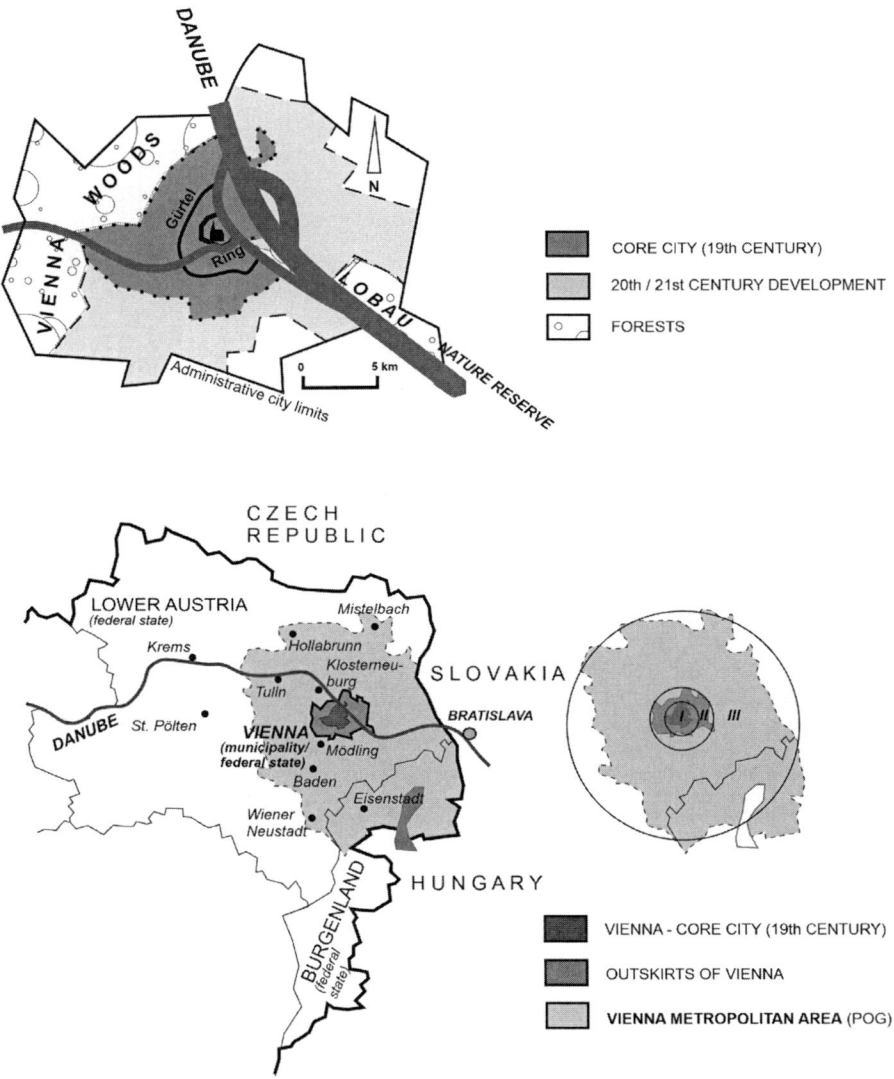

Fig. 1: Vienna: core city and metropolitan area (Illustration: Barbara Rief Vernay)

Suburbanisation in the form of single-family houses did not start until the 1960s, and thus later than in France, Germany, or the USA. The main reasons for out-migration from the core city were the poor condition of 19th century buildings and the declining quality of life due to the growing motorisation of urban traffic. At the same time, rising prosperity and the increasing popularity of the automobile[10] further spurred desires for "living in the countryside." These trends were met with large supplies of land reserves, low land prices, and newly created transport infrastructures in sought-after areas in Lower Austria. Suburbanisation was initially concentrated along the southbound axis around Baden and Wiener Neustadt, to the north around Korneuburg and Mistelbach, to the east around Gänserndorf, towards municipalities west of the Vienna Woods, and somewhat later towards the federal province of Burgenland.

Until the beginning of the 1990s, the suburban population grew steadily, while Vienna's population decreased in size.[11] Since Austria's accession to the EU in 1995, however, the city of Vienna has again recorded clear increases; between 2001 and 2021, the population grew from 1.55 to 1.92 million, mainly due to immigration from abroad.[12] In 2019, the entire metropolitan area counted 2.9 million inhabitants,[13] corresponding to an increase by 10% over the past decade— 55% of which attributable to the city of Vienna and 45% to its suburban areas[14].

Suburban Vienna's demographic growth has been paralleled by an increase in economic performance.[15] From a regional planning perspective, however, these urbanisation trends must be seen in a critical light. Since the 1950s, the expansion of residential areas, shopping centres, industrial sites, and leisure facilities has been taking place without legally binding spatial planning guidelines, resulting in extremely space-consuming, disorganised, and scattered spatial structures.[16] The proportion of detached single-family homes with only one or two dwellings ranges between 90% and 97%[17] (Fig. 2, 3). Due to these dispersive processes of urbanisation, increases in traffic and urban sprawl, Austria loses some 20 hectares of land every day to construction projects. These figures put Austria at the top of Europe[18]. Sustainable development would require an upper limit of 2.5 hectares per day[19]. These developments are favored by various factors, such as the autonomy of municipalities regarding land use

---

[10] Hartl, "Wanderungsbewegungen an die Peripherie der Stadt Wien," 256–257
[11] Fassmann and Goergl, "Das Stadtumland," 119.
[12] City of Vienna, "Integrationsmonitor 2020."
[13] Ringler et al., "Wohnen und Leben in der Stadtregion+."
[14] PGO (Planungsgemeinschaft Ost).
[15] Hartl, "Wanderungsbewegungen an die Peripherie der Stadt Wien," 254.
[16] Fassmann and Goergl, "Das Stadtumland," 127.
[17] Görgl et al., *Monitoring der Siedlungsentwicklung in der Stadtregion+ Wien: Strategien zur Räumlichen Entwicklung der Ostregion*, 78.
[18] „Boden und Bodenschutz - Situation in Österreich und in der EU, Factsheet 1/17", 2.
[19] Umweltbundesamt.

and construction regulations, but also subsidies from the public sector, including financial assistance for new construction projects or commuter allowances. Any disproportionate growth in suburban areas prompted by events such as the COVID-19 pandemic would also need to be evaluated in this light.

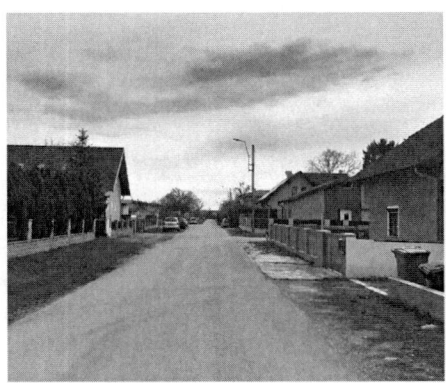 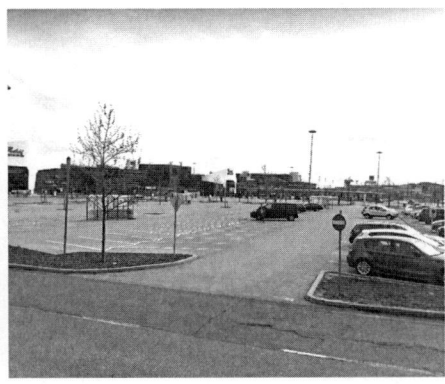

Fig. 2: Urban sprawl: Strasshof an der Nordbahn (Photo: Barbara Rief Vernay)

Fig. 3: Space-consuming urban development: large parking spaces at Shopping City Süd in the southern part of the commuter belt (Photo: Barbara Rief Vernay)

The COVID-19 pandemic and population trends in the suburban area

Since the onset of the pandemic, flight from the cities to nearby rural areas has received worldwide media attention, and numerous studies have been conducted to verify the hypothesis of pandemic-induced urban flight. Thus, a report by the Federal Reserve Bank of Cleveland has observed increased outward movements from New York for the period 2020/21,[20] a study by the Department of Geography and Planning of the University of Liverpool has described similar developments for British cities[21], a study by the French *Réseau Rural Français* confirmed

---

[20] Withaker, "Did the COVID-19 Pandemic Cause an Urban Exodus?."
[21] Rowe et al., "Urban exodus? Understanding human mobility in Britain during the COVID-19 pandemic using Meta-Facebook data."

increased migration out of Paris[22], and an article published in *Population, Space and Place* describes the same phenomenon for Spain[23]. However, these studies also suggest that, whereas above-average urban flight occurred in the early stages of the pandemic, the departure of residents is returning to pre-pandemic levels some two years later. The French and Spanish studies also indicate that the outward migration has not structurally changed urban areas as such and that these will continue to be poles of attraction, regardless of disease outbreaks or other crises.

Austrian media have discussed the phenomenon of urban flight in connection with the simultaneous growth of the suburban belt of Vienna. Thus, the state news channel ORF, in its report *The Pandemic and the Wealthy Beltway*, suggested that the COVID-19 pandemic had led to increased urban flight to suburban zones.[24] The daily newspaper *Der Standard* surmised that the pandemic would increase the suburbanisation phenomenon, simply because work, in times of digitalisation, was no longer bound to any one physical location.[25] Another daily, *Die Presse*, likewise expected the pandemic to push more people out of the cities,[26] hypothesizing that especially the suburban belt was going to gain population.[27] The most cited reason for out-migration was the desire for more open and green spaces as well as for more living space.

We are now going to examine to what extent the pandemic has indeed induced urban flight and will attempt to answer two questions: 1) Did the pandemic cause more people than before to move to suburban areas to escape the densely built-up city, and has the pandemic changed the population dynamics in suburban areas? 2) Has the pandemic noticeably changed the demand for housing and the prices for real estate in suburban areas?

Has the pandemic driven people out of the city?

To answer the first question, we traced the demographic developments in all of the suburban municipalities located within the boundaries of the Vienna metropolitan area for the period from 2012 to 2022. The figures used derive from the Central Register of Residents and include all persons who had been principally resident

---

[22] Rousseau, Collet and Delage, "Exode urbain: impacts de la pandémie de COVID-19 sur les mobilités résidentielles."
[23] González-Leonardo et al., "Understanding patterns of internal migration during the COVID-19 pandemic in Spain," 10.
[24] Schober, "Die Pandemie und der Speckgürtel."
[25] Lobe, "Ortlose Gesellschaft. Stadtflucht: Wer braucht noch Orte?."
[26] Fabry, "Stadtflucht und Home-Office werden nicht verschwinden."
[27] Metzler-Andelberg, "Landzuflucht de luxe. Der Speckgürtel von Wien legt wieder zu."

in a given municipality for more than 90 days as provided by the federal statistics office, *Statistik Austria*.[28] The growth curves presented are likewise based on data provided by *Statistik Austria*.

Out-migration from Vienna

Out-migration from Vienna has increased slightly since 2017. For example, in 2021 about 80,000 people left the city, with half of these moving abroad and most of the remainder (71%) distributed between the federal provinces of Lower Austria and Burgenland. However, these out-migration figures have been more than compensated for by immigration and positive birth rates, resulting in population growth in the pandemic years 2020 and 2021. The slightly decelerated growth between 2020 and 2021 compared to previous years is thought to be due to excess mortality caused by COVID-19 and a pandemic-related deceleration of immigration from abroad (Fig. 4).[29]

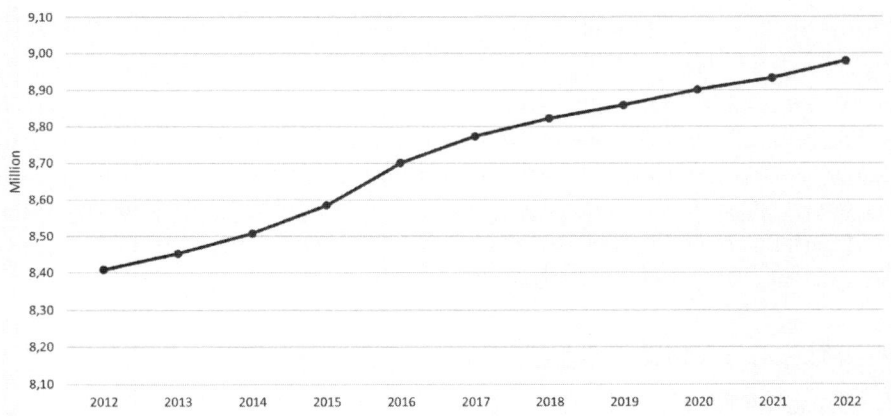

Fig. 4: City of Vienna, population development, 2012 to 2022
(Illustration: Barbara Rief Vernay)

---

[28] Statistics Austria, "Population at Beginning of Year/Quarte."
[29] City of Vienna, "Bevölkerungsentwicklung 2020: Wien wächst moderat weiter."

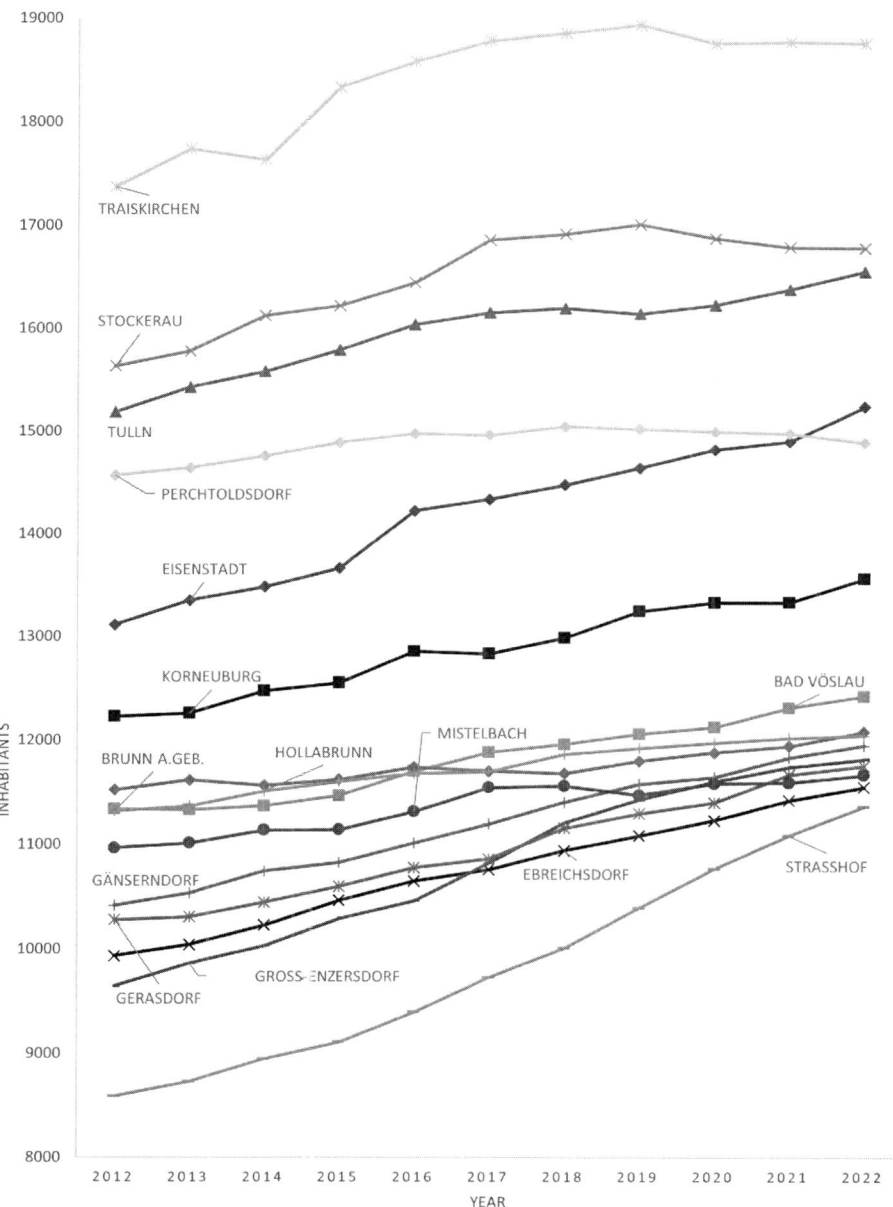

Fig. 5: Vienna metropolitan area: population development of selected communities, 2012 to 2022 (Illustration: Barbara Rief Vernay)

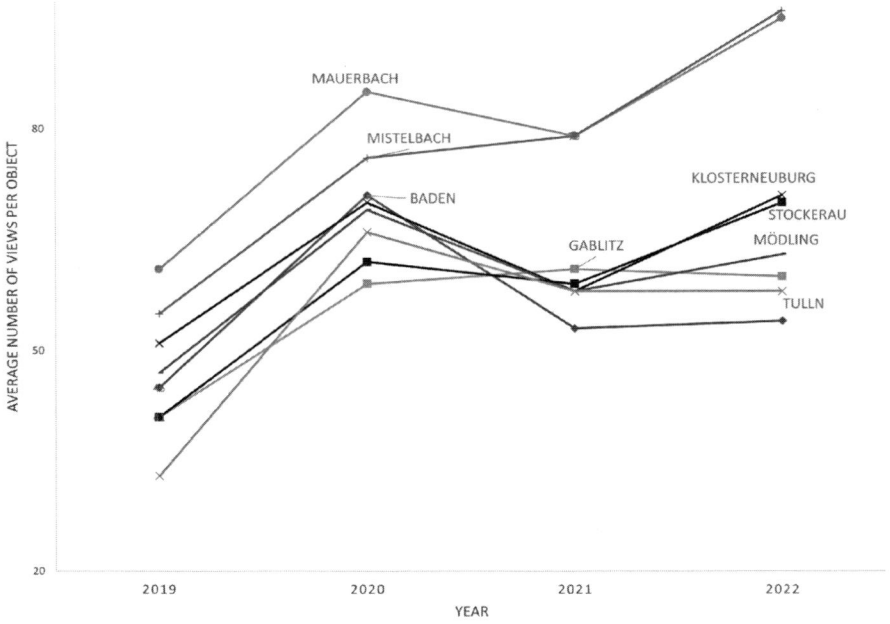

Fig.6: Development of queries for housing (2019 to 2022), selected communities around Vienna (Illustration: Barbara Rief Vernay)

Population growth in the municipalities of the suburban belt

Most of the 268 suburban municipalities have been growing steadily since annual recording began in 2002, with municipalities with fewer than 5,000 inhabitants showing the highest gains in population.[30] The most populous of these municipalities are located in the southern and northern parts of the suburban area. Only 5 of these have over 20,000 inhabitants (i.e., Klosterneuburg, Mödling, Baden, Schwechat, Wiener Neustadt), and they have not witnessed any noticeable deviations from prepandemic trends. The same is true for the 15 municipalities with a population size of 10,000 to 20,000 inhabitants (Fig. 5). In terms of population growth, 3 of these 15 municipalities have stagnated since 2019, while the remaining 12 have witnessed substantial increases that had started well before the pandemic. Of the 27 municipalities with 5,000 to 10,000 inhabitants, 5 have seen slight decreases in growth since 2020, 3 have seen slight decreases in population,

---

[30] Note: Population at the beginning of the year by municipalities, 2002 to 2022 (Statistics Austria).

and 8 have witnessed minor increases since 2021. Overall, however, these changes do not differ substantially compared to prepandemic times.

Of the 30 municipalities with 3,500 to 5,000 inhabitants, 3 have shown slight population decreases since 2020, while the rest have seen a slow but steady growth similar to that in the prepandemic era. Of the 72 municipalities with 2,000 to 3,500 inhabitants, 14 have decreased and the rest have increased in size, but again without substantial differences compared to before the pandemic. In the remaining 119 municipalities, whose population sizes range between 1,500 and 100, no significant changes have been seen since the start of the pandemic. Looking at the growth curves of municipalities not by size but by district, no notable changes have occurred since the start of the pandemic.

The data series of the municipalities surrounding Vienna show that the pandemic has not yet directly affected the population dynamics in the immediate vicinity of Vienna, i. e., it has, so far, not caused an extraordinary exodus of the Viennese population to surrounding municipalities—a finding that is in line with those seen in other urban regions in the world as outlined above. Of note, however, the residential registration data given above do not include people who moved to the countryside while still being registered in Vienna or those having taken up a secondary residence outside of Vienna.

Housing demand in suburban areas and deficits of the core city

The results presented above include actual migration movements only and do not reflect people's intention to move to suburban areas. Such information, however, is highly relevant in the pandemic context, because it provides indications on possible future migration flows from the city to suburbia.

Evolution of housing demand and real estate prices

To assess people's intention to move, we analysed the evolution of queries for housing based on data provided by *findmyhome.at* and *willhaben.at*, two of Austria's largest online real estate platforms.[31] Data include the numbers of available objects (i. e., apartments and houses) for sale per municipality per year and both the total and average numbers of views per municipality per year. Specifically, we asked whether online searches for real estate in suburban municipalities have increased since the beginning of the pandemic. The trends that emerge from the data are

---

[31] Findmyhome.at (09. 09. 2022, data on file), Willhaben.at (28. 02. 2023, data on file)

very similar for both internet platforms. Fig. 6, based on selected examples in the Vienna environs, depicts the average of both data sources.[32]

As expected, the results in terms of interest differ from data on actual migration. Obviously, an internet query is much easier to perform than a move, which requires substantial financial and logistical resources. Thus, queries for real estate in suburban areas increased by about 50% in 2020 compared to 2019. Interestingly, search requests rose to a similar extent across all municipalities as illustrated in Fig. 6 based on selected examples in the Vienna environs.

In 2020, the year the pandemic started, interest in housing and real estate increased sharply in municipalities such as Mauerbach, Klosterneuburg, Stockerau, and Mistelbach north of Vienna, Purkersdorf, Gablitz, and Tulln west of Vienna, and Mödling and Baden south of Vienna. In 2021, interest in these municipalities declined again (one exception being Gablitz), but remained above 2019 levels. While the 2021 drop in demand may have been due to the nationwide relaxation of COVID-19 measures, the renewed increase in interest in suburban-belt housing between 2021 and 2022 contradicts this assumption, it may even indicate a continued uptick in demand. This is also supported by the sharp rise in real estate prices.

The data also show that, since the beginning of the pandemic, the search for real estate has extended to zones that had previously been in lower demand due to their greater distances from Vienna. Examples include the municipalities of Krems (20% increase) and St. Pölten (60% increase), which are located 80 km and 65 km from Vienna, respectively. Both municipalities are situated outside the Vienna metropolitan area as defined by PGO. The increasing demand for these more distant locations may be related to a decreasing supply of available properties in Vienna's closer vicinities.

At the same time, whereas demand for housing properties in the core zone of Vienna has declined by about 25%, demand for properties with private open spaces (balcony, terrace, garden) has increased by 42%. It merits mention, however, that the supply of properties with private open spaces in Vienna is infinitely lower than in the surrounding suburban areas.

The increased demand for housing in the city's environs is reflected in the price trend. While real-estate prices outside the city limits are still, on average, about one third lower than within city limits,[33] they have risen at an above-av-

---

[32] Findmyhome, "Nachfrageentwicklung-Speckgürtel."
[33] Metzler-Andelberg, "Landzuflucht de luxe. Der Speckgürtel von Wien legt wieder zu."

erage rate since the pandemic. Before the pandemic, prices for single-family homes increased by 4.9% in Lower Austria and by 3.2% in Burgenland from 2018 to 2019[34]. In 2020, the corresponding increases were 7.4% and 8.9%, respectively[35], and in 2021, price increases even reached 11.3% and 13.7%, respectively[36]. Rental prices in Lower Austria and Burgenland have also risen since the start of the pandemic, but to a much lesser extent than purchase prices.[37]

Deficits of the 19th century city

The strong increase in demand for housing in suburban municipalities during the first two years of the pandemic may provide indications for future developments in the Viennese suburban belt. It may, however, also be an indication of deficits of the core city.

Approximately 40% of Vienna's population lives in the densely inhabited 19th century area.[38] Thanks to a city-wide renewal policy and funds from the City of Vienna[39], large parts of the 19th century neighborhoods in the core city have been successively redeveloped since the early 1970s.[40] Today, they are characterised by a use-variable, small-scale, socially mixed structure, with their layout allowing distances to be comfortably covered on foot or by bicycle, while offering a historic urban atmosphere.

Yet, these 19th century areas are still today facing urban planning problems. Thus, some neighbourhoods have very high building densities[41], such as areas around the *Gürtel* boulevard. With up to more than 500 inhabitants per hectare, they house four times the population of the city centre with 100 to 300 inhabitants per hectare[42]. At the same time, most of these densely populated areas lack green spaces. 19th century buildings are very rarely equipped with balconies, terraces, or gardens (Fig. 7). In addition, these historic zones lack public green space. Although 50% of Vienna's administrative urban area

---

[34] Statistics Austria, *Housing 2020, Figures, data and indicators of housing statistics,* 57.
[35] Ibid., 77.
[36] Ibid., 69.
[37] Ibid., 39, 54 and 48.
[38] City of Vienna, "Masterplan Gründerzeit, Handlungsempfehlungen zur qualitätsorientierten Weiterentwicklung der gründerzeitlichen Bestandsstadt", 18.
[39] Wiener Altstadterhaltungsfonds 1972, "Schutzzonen."
[40] Hatz and Lippl, "Stadterneuerung: Neues Wohnen in alten Quartieren," 148.
[41] Residential densities today vary between 200 and 500 persons per ha (City of Vienna, "Karte EinwohnerInnendichte 2020.").
[42] Stadt Wien, MA 18, Stadtentwicklung und Stadtplanung, Bevölkerungsevidenz April 2020, Realnutzungskartierung 2018, MA 01, MA 41

consists of green areas, these are unevenly distributed. The majority of them are situated in the northwestern and southeastern outskirts of the city, while the 19th century areas, especially those near *Gürtel,* have few planted areas within walking distance. High population concentrations with a simultaneous lack of public green spaces posed a particular problem during the pandemic curfews.

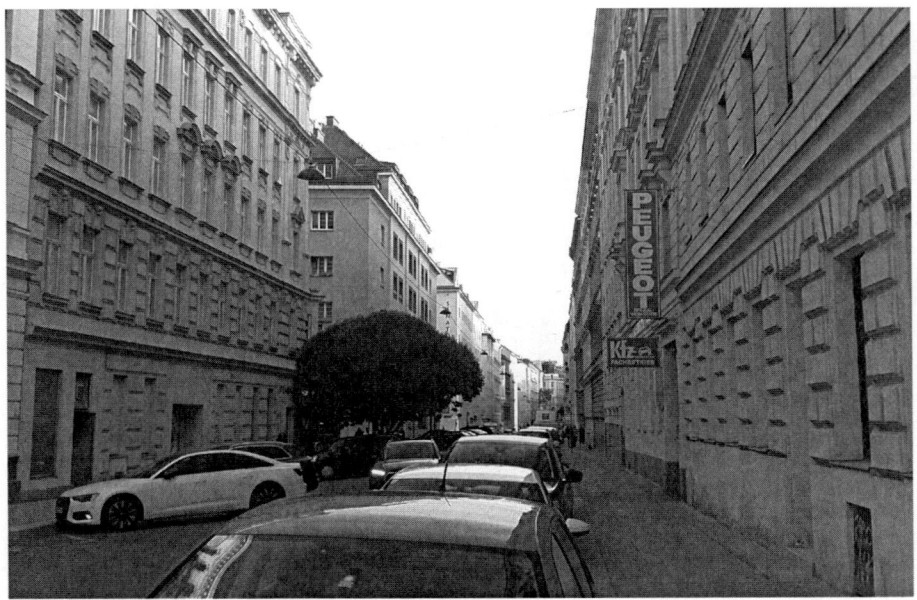

Fig.7: Typical street in the late 19th century built-up area (Photo: Barbara Rief Vernay)

In late 2020, the Department of Urban Planning of the City of Vienna drafted a technical paper[43] in response to the new urban planning challenges related to the COVID-19 crisis. It stated, among other things, that, in situations of crisis, it was necessary to focus on short- and medium-term strategies, such as the flexible use of public spaces. Yet, long-term objectives, such as a climate-friendly urban development, remained equally valid, because these are considered the basis for resilient urban structures. The paper also concluded

---

[43] Häberlin et al., "Corona: Die Rolle der Stadtplanung für die Krisenbewältigung am Beispiel Wien."

that 'density' should be considered an advantage, because only a certain density of facilities and service offerings – as is the case in polycentrically structured Vienna – ensures optimal supply networks in times of crisis.

Conclusion

The phenomenon of pandemic-induced urban flight was prominently discussed by news and media outlets around the world. Media across Austria assumed that, triggered by the pandemic and thanks to novel digital possibilities, increasing numbers of people would leave the densely populated areas of Vienna to move to rural-like areas outside the city and that urban flight would gain momentum, further exacerbating the problem of urban sprawl.

The results of this study indicate that, although the examined suburban areas have been experiencing a steady growth in population, growth curves have not changed noticeably two years after the start of the pandemic. We therefore assume that the pandemic has, so far, not influenced the demographic growth of Vienna's surrounding municipalities.

We also showed that interest in and demand for housing outside the core city of Vienna has risen sharply since the pandemic. The increased desire of the urban population to move out of the city is reflected by an increase in corresponding search queries on real-estate platforms. Only the coming years will show whether the desire to move will actually materialise. Of note, events such as economic or energy crises, changes in spatial planning guidelines, and modified public funding conditions are further factors influencing migration flows between the core city and the suburban belt.

Despite the changes we describe, the city of Vienna remains the most sought-after area in the entire metropolitan area, just as it was before the pandemic. Throughout the pandemic years, Vienna recorded an extraordinary increase in population and, thus, retained its supraregional appeal. For Vienna, increased migration to suburban areas by no means signifies suburbanisation in the sense of desertification and decay of the core city. At the same time, however, the pandemic crisis has revealed some of the deficits of Vienna's core city and has made the need for short-term and flexible urban planning strategies all the clearer.

Bibliography

"Boden und Bodenschutz – Situation in Österreich und in der EU, Factsheet 1/17." Accessed September 13, 2022. https://www.eu-umweltbuero.at/assets/Uploads/2021-2-Boden-und-Bodenschutz-in-der-EU.pdf.

Der Standard. "Wien Verliert ‚Economist'-Titel als lebenswerteste Stadt." June 9, 2021. Accessed September 12, 2021. https://www.derstandard.at/story/2000127248067/wien-verliert-economist-titel-als-lebenswerteste-stadt.

City of Vienna. "Bevölkerungsentwicklung 2020: Wien wächst Moderat Weiter." Accessed September 13, 2022. https://www.wien.gv.at/statistik/bevoelkerung/entwicklung-2020.html.

City of Vienna. "Integrationsmonitor 2020." Accessed September 15, 2022. https://www.wien.gv.at/spezial/integrationsmonitor2020/demografie-und-einwanderungsrecht/entwicklung-der-wiener-bevoelkerung-seit-1961/.

City of Vienna. "Karte EinwohnerInnendichte 2020." https://www.wien.gv.at/stadtentwicklung/grundlagen/stadtforschung/karten/bevoelkerung.html.

City of Vienna. "Masterplan Gründerzeit, Handlungsempfehlungen zur Qualitätsorientierten Weiterentwicklung der gründerzeitlichen Bestandsstadt." Werkstattbericht 180. Accessed September 20, 2022. https://www.digital.wienbibliothek.at/urn/urn:nbn:at:AT-WBR-579168

City of Vienna. *Realnutzungskartierung 2018.*

City of Vienna. *Stadtentwicklung Und Stadtplanung, Bevölkerungsevidenz April 2020.*

Fabry, Clemens. "Corona Kostet Wien den Titel ‚Lebenswerteste Stadt'." June 9, 2021. Accessed September 12, 2022. https://www.diepresse.com/5990955/corona-kostet-wien-den-titel-lebenswerteste-stadt.

Fabry, Clemens. "Stadtflucht und Home-Office werden nicht verschwinden." *Die Presse*, June 15, 2021. Accessed September 8, 2022. https://www.diepresse.com/5993292/stadtflucht-und-home-office-werden-nicht-verschwinden.

Fassmann, Heinz, and Peter Görgl. "Das Stadtumland." In *Wien: Städtebauliche Strukturen und gesellschaftliche Entwicklungen*. Edited by Gerhard Hatz, Walter Matznetter and Heinz Fassmann, 117–44. Wien, Köln, Weimar: Böhlau, 2009.

Findmyhome. "Nachfrageentwicklung-Speckgürtel." Accessed September 9, 2022. (Data on file).

González-Leonardo, Miguel, Antonio López-Gay, Niall Newsham, Joaquín Recaño, and Francisco Rowe. "Understanding Patterns of Internal Migration During the COVID-19 Pandemic in Spain." *Population, space and place* 28, no. 6 (2022). Accessed September 17, 2022. https://doi.org/10.1002/psp.2578.

Görgl, Peter, Heinz Fassmann, Jakob Eder, and Elisabeth Gruber. *Monitoring der Siedlungsentwicklung in der Stadtregion+: Strategien zur Räumlichen Entwicklung der Ostregion*. PGO (Planungsgemeinschaft OST), 2017. https://doi.org/10.13140/RG.2.2.26289.07525.

Hartl, Gerda. "Wanderungsbewegungen an Die Peripherie Der Stadt Wien." In *Wien – Budapest: Stadträume Des 20. Jahrhunderts Im Vergleich*. Edited by Máté Tamáska and Barbara Rief, 253–69. Vienna: Praesens, 2020.

Hatz, Gerhard, and Clemens Lippl. "Stadterneuerung: Neues Wohnen in alten Quartieren." In *Wien: Städtebauliche Strukturen Und Gesellschaftliche Entwicklungen*. Edited by Gerhard Hatz, Walter Matznetter and Heinz Fassmann, 147–79. Wien, Köln, Weimar: Böhlau, 2009.

Häberlin, Udo, Gerlinde Mückstein, Nils Peters, Gregor Stratil-Sauer, Johannes Suitner, Tobias Troger, and Maria Wasserburger. "Corona: Die Rolle Der Stadtplanung für Die Krisenbewältigung Am Beispiel Wien." In *REAL CORP 2020: Shaping Urban Change – Livable City Regions for the 21st Century: Proceedings of the 25th International Conference on Urban Planning, Regional Development and Information Society 15-18 September 2020, Virtual Conference = Beiträge zur 25. Internationalen Konferenz zu Stadtplanung, Regionalentwicklung und Informationsgesellschaft*. Edited by Manfred Schrenk et al. 2nd edition, 1271–81. Vienna: CORP – Competence Center of Urban and Regional Planning, 2020.

Lindenthal, Thomas, and Martin Schlatzer. *Risiken Für Die Lebensmittelversorgung in Österreich Und Lösungsansätze Für Eine Höhere Krisensicherheit: Diskussionspapier des Zentrums für globalen Wandel und Nachhaltigkeit*. Vienna: Universität für Bodenkultur, 2020. Accessed September 12, 2022. https://boku.ac.at/fileadmin/data/H01000/H10090/H10400/H10420/Lindenthal_und_Schlatzer_2020_Lebensmittelversorgung_und_Krisensicherheit.pdf.

Lobe, Adrian. "Ortlose Gesellschaft. Stadtflucht: Wer Braucht noch Orte?" *Der Standard*. Accessed September 12, 2022. https://www.derstandard.at/story/2000136427260/stadtflucht-wer-braucht-noch-orte.

Mezler-Andelberg, Sabine. "Landzuflucht De Luxe. Der Speckgürtel Von Wien Legt wieder zu." February 9, 2021. https://www.diepresse.com/5933523/der-speckguertel-von-wien-legt-wieder-zu.

PGO (Planungsgemeinschaft Ost). Accessed September 13, 2022. https://www.planungsgemeinschaft-ost.at/die-region/stadtregion.

Platzer, Monika. "Wien, Ein Sonderfall im 'Kalten Krieg'?" In *Wien – Budapest: Stadträume Des 20. Jahrhunderts Im Vergleich*. Edited by Máté Tamáska and Barbara Rief, 67–85. Vienna: Praesens, 2020.

Rainer, Roland. *Planungskonzept Wien. Der Aufbau 13*. Jugend & Volk, 1962.

Ringler, Paul, Bernhard Hoser, Günther Ogris, and David Laumer. *Wohnen und Leben in Der Stadtregion+: Endbericht Zur Studie*. Vienna, 2020. Accessed September 13, 2022. https://www.planungsgemeinschaft-ost.at/fileadmin/root_pgo/Studien/Raumordnung/Leben_und_Wohnen_in_der_Sadtregion__Analysebericht.pdf.

Rousseau, Max, Anaïs Collet, and Aurélie Delage. *Exode urbain: impacts de la pandémie de COVID-19 sur les mobilités résidentielles.*, 2022. Study by Réseau Rural Français. Accessed September 17, 2022. https://www.reseaurural.fr/centre-de-ressources/documents/etude-exode-urbain-impacts-pandemie.

Rowe, Francisco, Alessia Calafiore, Daniel Arribas-Bel, Krasen Samardzhiev, and Martin Fleischmann. "Urban Exodus? Understanding Human Mobility in Britain During the COVID-19 Pandemic Using Meta-Facebook Data." *Population, space and place* 29, no. 1 (2023). https://doi.org/10.1002/psp.2637.

Schober, Sandra. "Land statt Stadt. Die Pandemie und der Speckgürtel." *ORF*, September 7, 2021. Accessed September 8, 2022. https://orf.at/stories/3226288/.

Schrenk, Manfred, Vasily V. Popovich, Peter Zeile, Pietro Elisei, Clemens Beyer, Judith Ryser, Christa Reicher, and Canan Çelik, eds. *REAL CORP 2020: Shaping Urban Change - Livable City Regions for the 21st Century: Proceedings of the 25th International Conference on Urban Planning, Regional Development and Information Society 15-18 September 2020, Virtual Conference = Beiträge Zur 25. Internationalen Konferenz Zu Stadtplanung, Regionalentwicklung Und Informationsgesellschaft*. 2nd edition. Vienna: CORP - Competence Center of Urban and Regional Planning, 2020. https://conference.corp.at/fileadmin/proceedings/CORP2020_proceedings.pdf.

Statistic Austria. "Population at Beginning of Year/Quarte." Accessed September 13, 2022. https://www.statistik.at/statistiken/bevoelkerung-und-soziales/bevoelkerung/bevoelkerungsstand/bevoelkerung-zu-jahres-/-quartalsanfang.

Statistics Austria. *Housing 2020, Figures, Data and Indicators of Housing Statistics*. Vienna, 2018.

Umweltbundesamt. Accessed September 13, 2022. https://www.umweltbundesamt.at.

Whitaker, Stephan D. "Did the COVID-19 Pandemic Cause an Urban Exodus?." Cleveland Fed: District Data Briefs, February 5, 2021.

Wiener Altstadterhaltungsfonds 1972. *Schutzzonen*; (Altstadterhaltungsnovelle 1972; Landesgesetzblatt Nummer 16/1972).

Polarised Residential Preferences for the Centre and Outer Suburban Tokyo After the Experience of COVID-19

Keisuke Sakamoto, Takahiro Yamazaki, Toru Terada, Noriko Akita, Akito Murayama, Akiko Iida, Marco Amati, Makoto Yokohari

Introduction

For much of the 20th century Japan's urban and economic miracle has been understood as driven by a mixture of social and transportation networks, state sponsored industrialisation and agglomeration economies[1]. Similar to megacities internationally, Japanese ones have experienced a demographic movement known as the "back-to-the-city movement"[2] or "fifth migration"[3]. While Japanese urban populations have replicated suburbanisation trends in Europe and the U.S. between the 1960s and 90s[4,5], subsequent generations of these suburban migrants have migrated back to live in inner suburban locations for better services, opportunities and accessibility to the central business district (CBD)[6,7,8]. The back-to-the-city

---

[1] Hall, *Cities in Civilization 1999*, 455–456.
[2] Sturtevant and Jung, "Are we Moving Back to the City? Examining Residential Mobility in the Washington, DC Metropolitan Area."
[3] Fishman, "Longer View: The Fifth Migration."
[4] Champion, "Urban and Regional Demographic Trends in the Developed World."
[5] Sorensen, "Subcentres and Satellite Cities: Tokyo's 20th Century Experience of Planned Polycentrism."
[6] Lees, "Gentrification and Social Mixing: Towards an Inclusive Urban Renaissance?"
[7] Hyra, "The Back-to-the-City Movement: Neighbourhood Redevelopment and Processes of Political and Cultural Displacement."
[8] Schulz, "Trends of Revitalizing Central City Peripheries in Tokyo."

movement has brought with it a decline of outer suburban neighbourhoods[9,10,11], which, in the case of Tokyo, have been regarded as the frontline of an emerging megacity shrinkage owing to their poor access to the CBD and an ageing population[12,13].

However, the COVID-19 pandemic has drastically deprived residents of the freedom to commute and aggregate, while at the same time forcing an increased tolerance among businesses for working from home. A decline in the premium put on location and access has delivered a re-evaluation of residential environments in outer suburbs. Mouratidis[14] reviewed the pandemic's impacts on the relationships between cities and urban quality of life, arguing that citizens' preference for private mobility has risen[15,16], along with increased awareness of the walkability of neighbourhoods[17,18], access to blue or green spaces and nature[19,20], dwelling size and quality[21,22], and ICT infrastructure

---

[9] Phelps, Valler and Wood, "A Postsuburban World? An Outline of a Re-Search Agenda."
[10] Sweeney and Hanlon, "From Old Suburb to Post-Suburb: The Politics of Retrofit in the Inner Suburb of Upper Arlington, Ohio."
[11] Ohashi and Phelps, "Contrasts in Suburban Decline: A Tale of Three Key Outer Suburban 'Business Core Cities' in Tokyo Metropolis."
[12] Ohashi and Phelps, "Diversity in Decline: The Changing Suburban Fortunes of Tokyo Metropolis."
[13] Phelps and Ohashi, "Edge City Denied? The Rise and Fall of Tokyo's Outer Sub-Urban 'Business Core Cities'."
[14] Mouratidis, Kostas. "How COVID-19 Reshaped Quality of Life in Cities: A Synthesis and Implications for Urban Planning."
[15] Shakibaei et al., "Impact of the COVID-19 Pandemic on Travel Behavior in Istanbul: A Panel Data Analysis."
[16] Teixeira and Lopes, "The Link Between Bike Sharing and Subway Use During the COVID-19 Pandemic: The Case-Study of New York's Citi Bike."
[17] Finucane et al., "Do Social Isolation and Neighbourhood Walkability Influence Relationships Between COVID-19 Experiences and Wellbeing in Predominantly Black Urban Areas?"
[18] Oishi, Cha and Schimmack, "The Social Ecology of COVID-19 Cases and Deaths in New York City: The Role of Walkability, Wealth, and Race."
[19] Douglas et al., "Mitigating the Wider Health Effects of Covid-19 Pandemic Response."
[20] Ugolini et al., "Effects of the COVID-19 Pandemic on the Use and Perceptions of Urban Green Space: An International Exploratory Study."
[21] Lehberger et al., "Self-Reported Well-Being and the Importance of Green Spaces – a Comparison of Garden Owners and Non-Garden Owners in Times of COVID-19."
[22] Poortinga et al., "The Role of Perceived Public and Private Green Space in Subjective Health and Wellbeing During and After the First Peak of the COVID-19 Outbreak."

and systems[23,24]. Da Schio et al.[25] note through a Belgium case study that the COVID-19 pandemic has led residents without access to private green space to seek to move to a new residential location in a greener neighbourhood.

While city centre location and access can be supposed to remain as primary determinants of residential preference, it can be hypothesised that post COVID-19 residential preferences in megacities will become polarised in a tug-of-war between the attractions of the centre of the metropolis and outer suburban areas, as residents who are able to work from home can tolerate a longer commute on necessary occasions. The concentrated urban amenities of the centre might still appeal to a large population, but equally, the value of surrounding nature and spacious residence in outer suburbs will grow, particularly if ICT infrastructure enables work to occur in locations far from CBD offices. Meanwhile, this polarisation could raise new concerns for the depopulation of inner suburbs that have neither the advantages of close commuting distance from the CBD or natural amenity.

A polarisation of residential preference by location inside megacities can be identified by examining the relationship between citizens' residential preference and the following three socio-geographical factors: average land prices in a neighbourhood, municipal day-night ratio of population, and distance from the CBD. All three factors represent respectively the willingness to pay for proximity to services and jobs; the attraction of a location for work and commerce[26] and the cost in terms of time and money for travel. Assuming that urban attractions exert a pull effect on a considerable population after COVID-19, neighbourhoods that enjoy high land prices and large daytime population like central areas will still positively relate to residential preference. At the same time, a reappraisal of the benefits of a natural environment and the demand for more space in residences triggered by working from home during the pandemic is expected to generate a positive relationship between distance and preference in these locations. The hypothesised linear combination of urban attractions and natural attractions for residential preferences after COVID-19 can be represented as Fig. 1.

---

[23] Haas, Faber and Hamersma, "How COVID-19 and the Dutch 'Intelligent Lockdown' Change Activities, Work and Travel Behaviour: Evidence from Longitudinal Data in the Netherlands."
[24] Shamshiripour et al., "How Is COVID-19 Reshaping Activity-Travel Behavior? Evidence from a Comprehensive Survey in Chicago."
[25] Da Schio et al., "The Impact of the COVID-19 Pandemic on the Use of and Attitudes Towards Urban Forests and Green Spaces: Exploring the Instigators of Change in Belgium."
[26] Foley, "Urban Daytime Population: A Field for Demographic-Ecological Analysis."

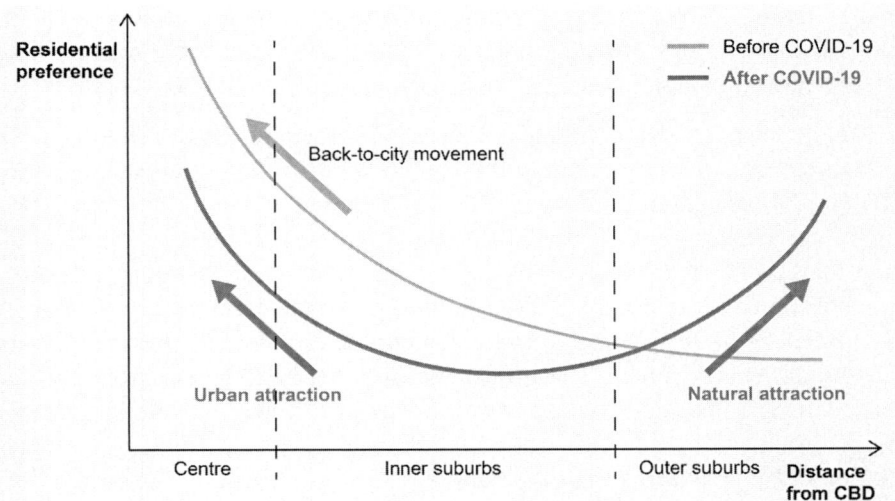

Fig. 1: Hypothetical diagram of polarised residential preference after COVID-19 according to suburban location (Illustration: Keisuke Sakamoto, Marco Amati, Makoto Yokohari)

The impacts of COVID-19 on residential preference are potentially varied, and there are a growing number of studies and reports that address the impacts of COVID-19 on urban residential preference and mobility. While some focused on the relationships according to individual socioeconomic attributes[27,28,29], and others have focused on housing preference[30,31], the influence of COVID-19 on the relation between residential preference and socio-geographical factors in municipalities and neighbourhoods have not yet been empirically verified. In particular, the identification of a trend towards polarised residential preferences between the centre and outer suburbs of a metropolis after the spread of COVID-19 is novel, compared to existing knowledge about a trend

---

[27] Jones and Grigsby-Toussaint, "Housing Stability and the Residential Context of the COVID-19 Pandemic."
[28] Devine-Wright et al., "'Re-Placed'- Reconsidering Relationships with Place and Lessons from a Pandemic."
[29] Pagani et al., "How the First Wave of COVID-19 in Switzerland Affected Residential Preferences."
[30] Zarrabi, Yazdanfar and Hosseini, "COVID-19 and Healthy Home Preferences: The Case of Apartment Residents in Tehran."
[31] Gür, "Post-Pandemic Lifestyle Changes and Their Interaction with Resident Behavior in Housing and Neighborhoods: Bursa, Turkey."

towards monocentric suburbanisation with a monotonic relationship between location preference and distance after the infection.

The planning, retrofit and future sustainability of megacities depends on gaining new insights about the relationship between socio-geographical factors and residential preferences, allowing the post-COVID-19 urban structural relationships to be better understood. Therefore, this study aims to verify the hypothesis that a polarised residential preference exists in Tokyo and demonstrates how this is affected by socio-geographical factors.

Study site

There are various definitions of the boundary of the Tokyo metropolitan area, but in the following we use Asakawa's[32] definition of the area including municipalities within a radius of 60 km from the central Tokyo business district. Using this definition, we can currently identify 202 municipalities belonging to the prefectures of Tokyo, Kanagawa, Saitama, Chiba, and Ibaraki (Fig. 2), where about 35 million people live. For an online survey explained below, the study site comprises 13 Japanese municipalities in the Tokyo metropolitan area that vary from central-metropolitan wards to a new town: Atsugi, Machida, Tama, Chofu, Mitaka, Musashino, Meguro, Shibuya, Koto, Matsudo, Koshigaya, Kashiwa, and Tsukuba. They are spread across Tokyo's metropolitan area in a belt roughly 100 kms long (Fig. 3). All of these sample municipalities have a population of more than 150,000, which allows for large enough sample populations. Furthermore, the selection of these targeted municipalities in a belt is expected to reduce variance of commuting routes or directions to CBD.

As mentioned in Sorensen[33], the suburbanisation of populations from the central areas of Tokyo including Meguro, Shibuya, and Koto progressed between the 1960s and 90s, and the inner suburban areas of Machida, Tama, Chofu, Mitaka, Musashino, Matsudo, and Kashiwa, enjoyed remarkable population growth, whereas the demographic change in the outer suburban area including Atsugi and Tsukuba was comparatively slow. After the bubble economy burst in the early 90s, however, central areas have increased in population again while urban populations have shrunk in outer suburban areas[34].

---

[32] Asakawa, "Changes in the Socio-Spatial Structure in the Tokyo Metropolitan Area: Social Area Analysis of Changes from 1990 to 2010."

[33] Sorensen, "Subcentres and Satellite Cities: Tokyo's 20th Century Experience of Planned Polycentrism."

[34] Ohashi and Phelps, "Contrasts in Suburban Decline: A Tale of Three Key Outer Suburban 'Business Core Cities' in Tokyo Metropolis."

The targeted 13 municipalities were divided into 873 neighbourhoods according to their zip codes (Fig. 4). A preliminary analysis shows that the neighbourhoods with a high population density lie mostly along the railway networks and the number of high-density neighbourhoods rapidly decreases beyond a distance of 30 km from CBD.

The first wave of the pandemic in Japan occurred around April 2020, and since then the number of infected people increased with an up-and-down fluctuation. Tokyo is the centre of the pandemic in Japan, and the government has intermittently declared a state of emergency in Tokyo four times since April 2020 in accordance with the rise of the wave of infections. These have required private urban facilities like restaurants or stores to shorten business hours or to close and have also included warnings to citizens not to go out except in an emergency. The number of infected people in the Tokyo metropolitan area has amounted to about 10,000 per day with the biggest wave in August 2021 at its peak followed by a rapid decrease to about 50 per day and temporarily subsiding in November.

Questionnaire survey

To examine the residential preference of citizens in the study areas, a questionnaire survey was conducted online. The survey included questions about demographic attributes including sex, age, zip code, length of residency, marital status, number of family members, daily use of a private car, and household income. Housing types were classified into the following eight categories: owner of a detached house, owner of a flat, rental of a detached house, rental of a flat, public housing, company housing, shared house, and others. Job types were also classified into the following six categories: private company employee, public servant, self-employed, freelance, temporary worker, and part-time employee. In addition, commuting conditions were identified by asking for workplace location and the frequency with which this changed to working from home or teleworking, before the spread of the infection (before January 2020) and during a pandemic period (from January to September 2021).

We then asked residents about their residential preference and whether they were willing to move to another neighbourhood due to the infection with the following four choices: "I have already moved," "I want to stay," "I have no idea," and "I want to move." Moreover, if they answered, "I have already moved," or "I want to move", we also asked whether they prefer to relocate to the inside or outside of the metropolitan area compared to their existing location to grasp how the infection has altered the target for their residential preferences. The online questionnaire was distributed to 44,660 persons in the 13 municipalities proportionally in accordance with each municipal population, and 7,996 of them (17.9%) answered from 16th to 18th November 2021 when the biggest wave of the pandemic at that time since July 2021 briefly subsided.

Data collection of socio-geographical factors

In addition to the individual variables gathered through the questionnaire survey, data on several socio-geographical factors of municipalities and neighbourhoods were also collected.

Socio-geographical factors were selected to identify a polarisation of residential preference. Using the latest official data provided by the government, these included the land price of the neighbourhood, the distance from the CBD, and municipal day-night ratio of population. Neighbourhood land price was constructed from the government database of the official land price, which is annually assessed by the municipalities using a standardised metric. The mean of the official land prices per m2 in 2019 was calculated in each neighbourhood as a representative value for the value of the respondent's land. The distance from CBD was represented by the distance from the centroid of a neighbourhood to Tokyo Station, which was calculated using ArcGIS 10.8 based on geospatial data. The municipal day-night ratio of population of each municipality was acquired by referring to data from national censuses, which have been officially conducted nationwide every five years to grasp the demographic and socio-economic condition of the population. This study utilised the statistics of 1995 and 2015.

Other basic socio-geographical data, specifically, the proportion of land-use zoning, population density, density of park catchment areas, forest density, and agricultural land density, were also collected from the latest government database and appropriately processed using ArcGIS 10.8 for the following analysis. The proportion of land-use zoning was classified into four categories: low residential area, tall residential area, commercial area, and industrial area. Population density was calculated according to the population in 2015 per area of each neighbourhood. Forest density and agricultural land density were also standardised by the area of each neighbourhood using forest and agricultural land data in 2015 aggregated on the basis of 100 m square grids. Catchment area density of the park was calculated by referring to an assumed catchment area used by the government, which for a small park (~0.25 ha) is 250 m radius circle, a medium park (~2.0 ha) is 500 m radius circle, and a large park (~4.0 ha) is 1,000 m radius circle, so the catchment area density of each park was calculated by the total sum of circle area for each neighbourhood in 2011. Catchment area for a multi-purpose city park is not assumed by the government, but

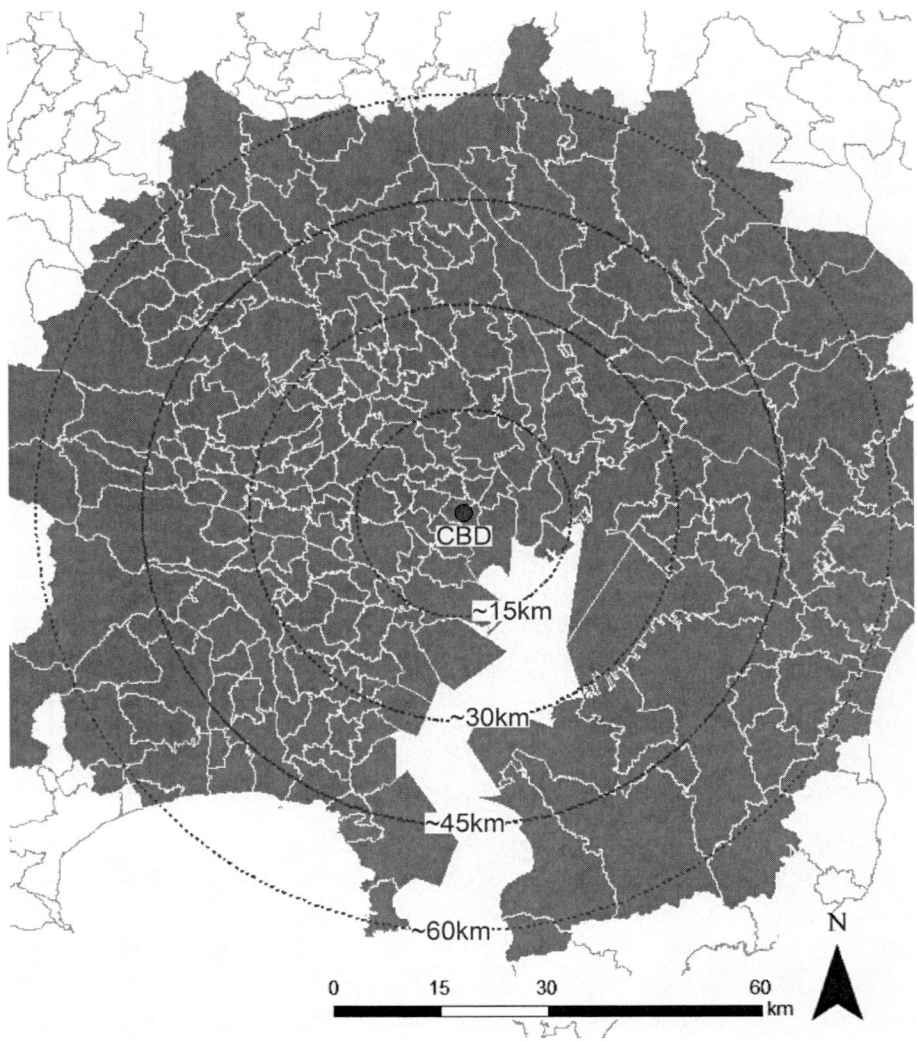

Fig. 2: Location of municipalities of the Tokyo metropolitan area
(Illustration: Keisuke Sakamoto, Marco Amati, Makoto Yokohari)

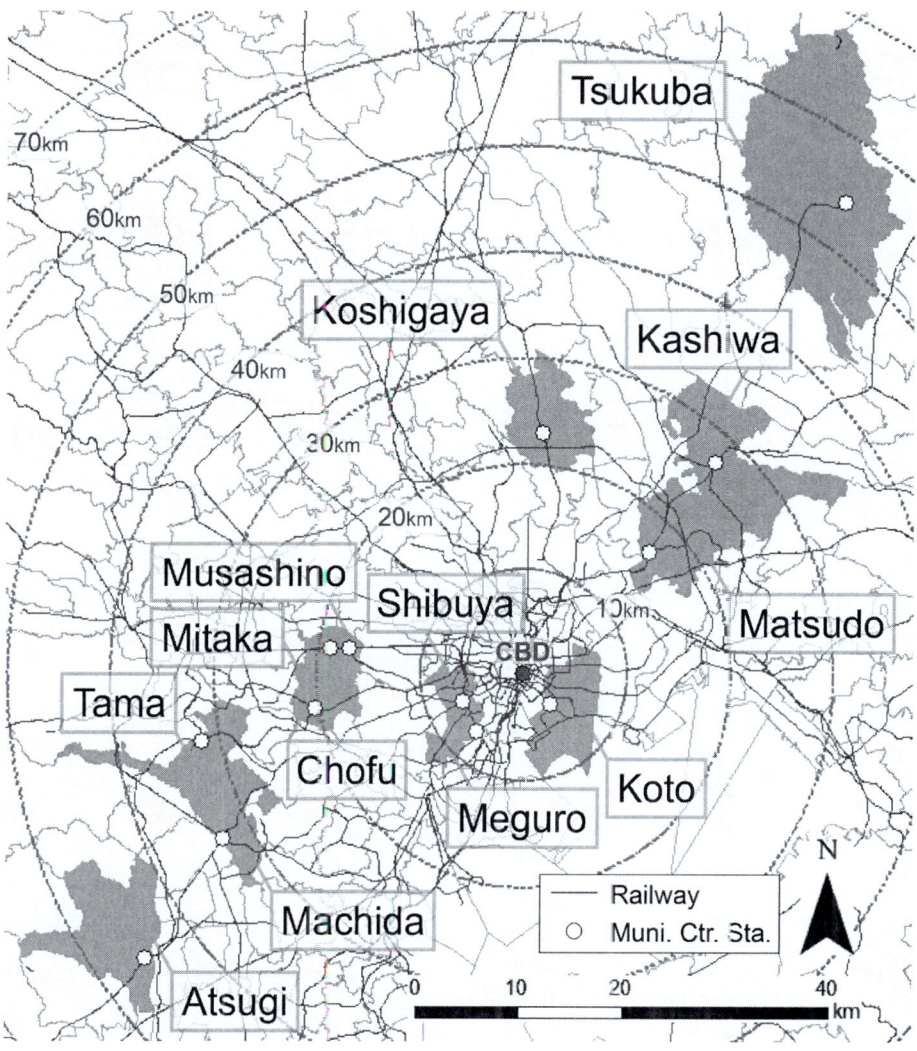

Fig. 3: Location of the study site
(Illustration: Keisuke Sakamoto, Marco Amati, Makoto Yokohari)

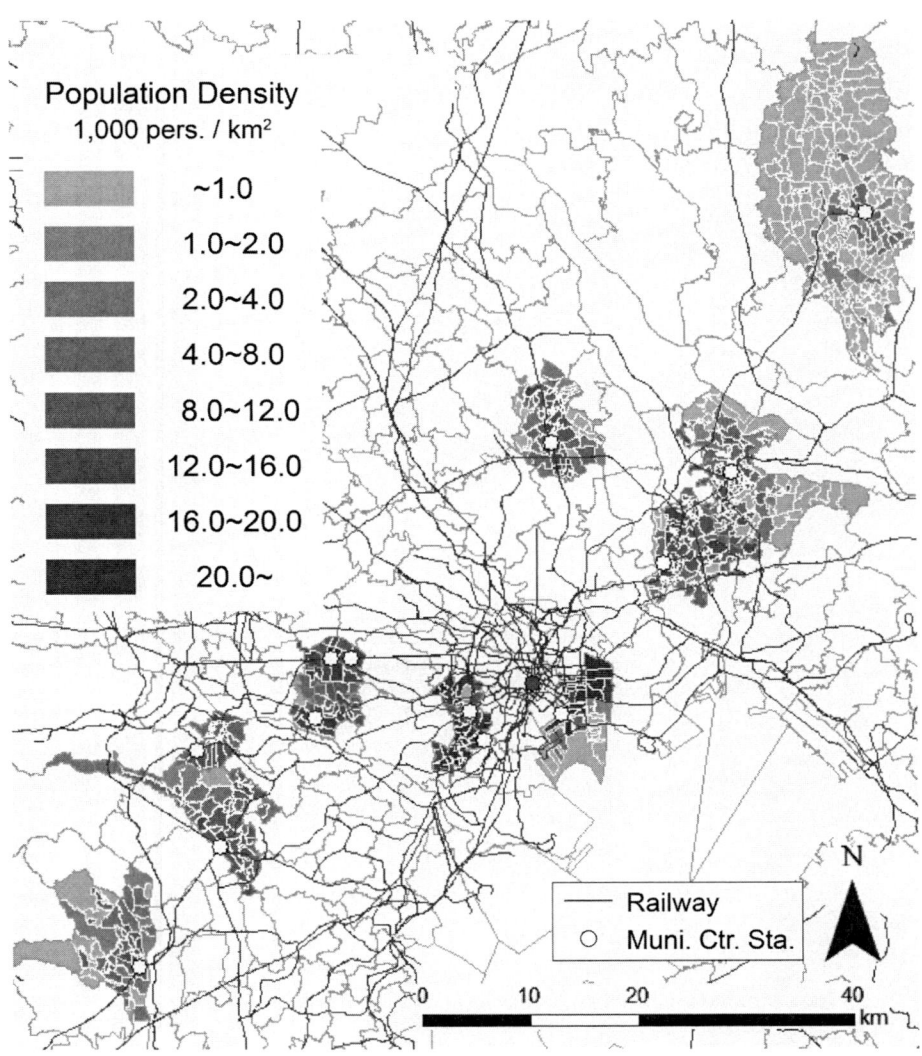

Fig. 4: Population density in the study site (Illustration: Keisuke Sakamoto, Marco Amati, Makoto Yokohari)

its size (>10 ha) is bigger than that of a large park (~4.0 ha), so catchment area was also set to 1,000 m radius circle as with a large park.

Analysis of residential preferences using ordinal logistic regression models

The relationships between residential preference after the experience of COVID-19 and the socio-geographical factors of municipalities and neighbourhoods were analysed using ordinal logistic regression analyses. Basic individual factors included sex, age, zip code, length of residency, marital status, number of family members, daily use of private car, household income, housing type, job type, commuting distance, and change in teleworking frequency per week. The household income was divided by the square root of the number of family members for standardisation. The commuting distance was represented by the distance between the centroid of the neighbourhood based on zip codes where the respondent lives and the centroid of the municipality where the workplace is located, which was calculated using ArcGIS 10.8. The individual factors were nested within neighbourhoods (zip codes), and furthermore, nested within the 13 municipalities. The neighbourhood-level factors included distance from the CBD to each neighbourhood, proportion of land-use zoning, population density, catchment area density of park, forest density, agricultural land density, and land price. The land price was converted into a logarithm assuming that it follows a lognormal distribution. The municipality-level factors included municipal ratio of day-night population in 2015, change in the ratio of day-night population between 1995 and 2015 standardised by the value for 1995.

The individual level factors and the neighbourhood and municipality level factors were arranged as explanatory variables in the multilevel analysis and the response variable, residential preference after the experience of COVID-19, was defined as an ordinal variable according to the answer in the questionnaire. If the answer was "I have already moved" or "I want to stay," this group seemed to express satisfaction with their neighbourhoods, if the answer was "I have no idea", this group was assumed to be expressing uncertainty of their relocation, and if the answer was "I want to move," these were considered to express dissatisfaction, and hence the three groups were valued at 2, 1, and 0 in order regarding their residential preference.

The individual variables are nested in neighbourhoods or municipalities, so there is a possibility to use multilevel regression analyses if the design effect (DEFF) between neighbourhood-level or municipality-level are more than

Response variable	Residential preference	"I have already moved": 222 (6.5%)
Individual level factors	N=3,439	
	Sex	Male: 2,324 (67.6%)
	Age (years old)	Mean: 50.9 (SD: 11.1)
	Length of residency (months)	Mean: 181.6 (SD: 150.5)
	Marriage	Yes: 2,113 (61.4%)
	Number of family members	Mean: 2.5 (SD: 1.2)
	Daily use of private car	Yes: 1,943 (56.5%)
	Family income (million yen/year)	~1.0: 56 (1.6%)
		4.0~5.0: 422 (12.3%)
		8.0~9.0: 249 (7.2%)
		15.0~20.0: 116 (3.4%)
	Housing type	Owner-occupied detached house: 1,285 (37.4%)
		Public housing: 126 (3.7%)
	Job type	Private company employee: 1,947 (56.6%)
		Temporary worker: 276 (8.0%)
	Commuting distance (km)	Mean: 13.1 (SD: 20.7)
	Change in teleworking frequency (/week)	Mean: 0.69 (SD: 2.0)
Neighbourhood level factors	N=417	
	Proportion of land-use zoning	Low residential: 34.0%
	Population density (/km2)	Mean: 1296.0 (SD: 676.0)
	Catchment area density of park (%)	Small park ... Mean: 98.0 (SD: 77.6)
	Agricultural land density (10^{-10}%)	Mean: 2.9 (SD: 6.6)
	Forest density (10^{-10}%)	Mean: 3.4 (SD: 7.2)
	Distance from CBD (km)	Mean: 22.0 (SD:12.4)
	Land price (thousand yen/m2)	Mean: 498.0 (SD:733.4)
Municipality level factors	N=13	
	Ratio of day-night population in 2015 (%)	Mean: 108.5 (SD:39.4)
	Change in ratio of day-night population between 1995 and 2015 (%)	Mean: 2.8 (SD:8.8)

Table 1: Basic statistics of variables for ordinal logistic regression analysis

2.0^{35}. Therefore, whether single-level analyses or multilevel analyses should be utilised is decided after calculating the DEFFs.

Basic statistics of target samples

Amongst all 7,996 respondents of the questionnaire survey, 3,439 live in 417 neighbourhoods of 13 municipalities (0.090% of the total population) complete with all the necessary variables for analyses, including 166 persons in Atsugi (0.074%), 350 in Machida (0.081%), 160 in Tama (0.109%), 284 in Chofu

---

[35] Muthen and Satorra, "Complex Sample Data in Structural Equation Modelling."

Response variable	"I want to stay": 2,510 (73.0%)	"I have no idea": 599 (17.4%)	"I want to move": 108 (3.1%)
Individual level factors			
	Female: 1,115 (32.4%)		
	No: 1,326 (38.6%)		
	No: 1,496 (43.5%)		
	1.0˜2.0: 102 (3.0%)	2.0˜3.0: 254 (7.4%)	3.0˜4.0: 361 (10.5%)
	5.0˜6.0: 374 (10.9%)	6.0˜7.0: 318 (9.2%)	7.0˜8.0: 322 (9.4%)
	9.0˜10.0: 285 (8.3%)	10.0˜12.0: 293 (8.5%)	12.0˜15.0: 198 (5.8%)
	20.0˜: 89 (2.6%)		
	Owner-occupied flat: 843 (24.5%)	Rental detached house: 46 (1.3%)	Rental flat: 1,048 (30.5%)
	Company housing: 58 (1.7%)	Share house: 18 (0.5%)	Others: 15 (0.4%)
	Public servant: 250 (7.3%)	Self-employed: 222 (6.5%)	Freelance: 147 (4.3%)
	Part-time employee: 597 (17.4%)		
Neighbourhood level factors			
	Tall residential: 38.1%	Commercial: 10.1%	Industrial: 17.8%
	Medium park ... Mean: 22.7 (SD: 36.4)	Large park ... Mean: 14.5 (SD: 28.5)	Multi-purpose park ... Mean: 43.9 (SD: 58.3)
Municipality level factors			

Table 1: Basic statistics of variables for ordinal logistic regression analysis

(0.124%), 229 in Mitaka (0.123%), 162 in Musashino (0.112%), 257 in Meguro (0.093%), 255 in Shibuya (0.114%), 447 in Koto (0.091%), 425 in Matsudo (0.088%), 227 in Koshigaya (0.067%), 351 in Kashiwa (0.085%), and 126 in Tsukuba (0.056%). The 417 neighbourhoods can be divided into 78 neighbourhoods (18.7%) in the three central wards, Shibuya, Meguro, and Koto, and 339 neighbourhoods (81.3%) in the other 10 suburban cities.

All the persons sampled were employed and therefore unemployed persons, homemakers, retirees or students were not included in the analysis. Basic statistics of target samples are displayed in Table 1. The ratio of males to females was almost 2:1. Ages of respondents were classified into 124 persons (3.61%)

≥20-29, 420 (12.2%) ≥30-39, 922 (26.8%) ≥40-49, 1,193 (34.7%) ≥50-59, 631 (18.4%) ≥60-69, 137 (3.98%) ≥70-79, and 12 (0.35%) ≥80-89. The ratio of the married to unmarried was nearly 3:2, and the number of family members was classified into 863 persons (25.1%) living alone, 1,088 (31.6%) living with two people, 769 (22.4%) with three, 520 (15.1%) with four, 153 (4.5%) with five, 29 (0.8%) with six, 13 (0.4%) with seven, and 4 (0.1%) with eight. The ratio of owner housing to rental housing was almost 3:2. Length of residency was classified into 1,447 persons (42.1%) for less than 10 years, 1,033 (30.0%) for between 10 and 19 years, 578 (16.8%) for between 20 and 29 years (27.1%), 191 (5.6%) for between 30 and 39 years, 107 (3.1%) for between 40 and 49 years, 54 (1.6%) for between 50 and 59 years, 26 (0.76%) for between 60 and 69 years, and 3 (0.09%) for more than 70 years. About 90% were employees, and other 10% were self-employed or freelance. Their commuting distance was classified into 1,265 persons (36.8%) within 5.0 km, 633 (18.4%) between 5.0 km and 10 km, 733 (21.3%) between 10 km and 20 km, 567 (16.5%) between 20 km and 30 km, 194 (5.6%) between 30 km and 50 km, and 47 (1.4%) beyond 50 km. Regarding change in teleworking frequency after the pandemic, 30% of all respondents had experienced increases in teleworking frequency, whereas no change had occurred to 60% and 10% had decreased their frequency.

The response variable, residential preference after the experience of COVID-19, was divided into ~80% comprising a satisfied group ("I have already moved" or "I want to stay"), ~17% as an uncertain group ("I have no idea"), and 3% as a dissatisfied group ("I want to move"). The three contextual factors related to the hypothesis of polarised residential preference, i.e. neighbourhood land prices, municipal day-night population ratios, and distance from CBD, were prepared as follows. The land prices of all 417 neighbourhoods were classified into 90 (21.6%) under 100,000 yen/m2, 160 (38.4%) between 100,000 and 200,000 yen/m2, 36 (8.6%) between 200,000 and 300,000 yen/m2, 38 (9.1%) between 300,000 and 500,000 yen/m2, and 93 (22.3%) over 500,000 yen/m2. The distance from the CBD for each neighbourhood was classified into 69 (16.6%) within 10 km, 58 (13.9%) between 10 km and 20 km, 158 (37.9%) between 20 km and 30 km, 57 (13.7%) between 30 km and 40 km, 47 (11.3%) between 40 km and 50 km, and 28 (6.7%) beyond 50 km. The 13 municipal day-night ratios of population in 2015 (and 1995) were 115.6% in Atsugi (119.4%), 91.7% in Machida (87.9%), 101.0% in Tama (82.6%), 86.4% in Chofu (85.3%), 88.7% in Mitaka (84.2%), 108.7% in Musashino (114.0%), 105.8% in Meguro (111.7%), 240.1% in Shibuya (285.2%), 122.2% in Koto (120.0%), 82.0% in Matsudo (76.2%), 87.3% in Koshigaya (79.0%), 90.4% in Kashiwa (83.7%), and 107.6% in Tsukuba (103.7%).

Residential preference influenced by the spread of COVID-19

City	Distance from Tokyo Station to the main station (km)	„I want to stay"	„I have already moved"		„I have no idea"	„I want to move"	
			To the inside of the metropolis	To the outside of the metropolis		To the inside of the metropolis	To the outside of the metropolis
Koto	3,91	72,04%	3,58%	0,22%	17,45%	2,24%	4,47%
Shibuya	6,89	66,67%	4,31%	0,39%	23,53%	1,18%	3,92%
Meguro	6,99	73,54%	5,45%	0,00%	13,62%	2,33%	5,06%
Matsudo	16,95	70,59%	1,88%	0,71%	19,29%	2,59%	4,94%
Musashino	18,82	64,20%	4,32%	1,23%	21,60%	3,09%	5,56%
Mitaka	20,72	76,86%	3,06%	0,00%	15,28%	2,18%	2,62%
Koshigaya	20,75	76,65%	0,00%	0,88%	16,74%	1,32%	4,41%
Chofu	22,39	71,48%	2,11%	0,70%	18,31%	3,52%	3,87%
Kashiwa	27,30	76,92%	1,42%	1,14%	12,54%	2,56%	5,41%
Tama	34,86	75,63%	2,50%	0,63%	18,75%	1,25%	1,25%
Machida	34,91	72,57%	1,14%	1,14%	17,43%	2,57%	5,14%
Atsugi	46,94	77,11%	0,60%	0,60%	19,28%	0,00%	2,41%
Tsukuba	52,86	78,57%	0,79%	2,38%	13,49%	3,17%	1,59%
Mean	**24,18**	**72,99%**	**2,44%**	**0,70%**	**17,42%**	**2,24%**	**4,22%**

Table 2: Residential preference influenced by the spread of COVID-19

Table 2 shows the residential preference influenced by the spread of COVID-19 based on the answers of the online questionnaire survey targeting the 13 municipalities in order of the distance from Tokyo Station to the main station of each municipality. The mean proportion of those who changed their residential preference due to the spread of COVID-19 ("I have already moved" or "I want to move") is 9.60%, which suggests that about 10% of people in the Tokyo metropolitan area have changed their original residential preference because of the effects of COVID-19 and they have been considering or have already relocated. Out of the other 90%, 73% have maintain their original residential preference ("I want to stay"), but 17% have expressed uncertainty in their future residential preference ("I have no idea"). The mean proportion of those who have shown satisfaction with their residential location ("I want to stay" or "I have already moved") is 76.13%, and the maximum proportion is 81.74% of Tsukuba, while the minimum proportion is 69.76% of Musashino.

Fig. 5, 6, and 7 indicate the relations between the residential preferences influenced by the spread of COVID-19 and the distance from the central Tokyo business districts to the main station of each of 13 targeted municipalities. Fig. 5 shows that the closer the municipality is to Tokyo Station, the more people have moved to the inside of the metropolis (R=0.712, p<0.01), while the more distant the municipality is from Tokyo Station, the more people have moved to the outside (R=0.680, p=0.011). The total proportion of those two groups increases proportionally to the proximity of Tokyo Station (R=0.526, p=0.065), and therefore actual relocation has been likely to proceed more towards the inside of the metropolis than the outside.

However, Fig. 6, which shows the relations between the proportion of "I want to move" due to COVID-19, identifies that the closer the municipality is to Tokyo Station, the more people are willing to move to other municipalities (R=0.592, p=0.033), and especially, people living in the inside of the metropolis exhibit a preference for the outside (R=0.480, p=0.097). Furthermore, the proportion of those who wish to remain in place even after COVID-19 answering "I want to stay" increase as the municipality increases in distance from Tokyo Station (R=0.579, p=0.038) (Fig. 7), which indicates that the closer the municipality is to the Tokyo Station, the more likely people are to prefer a new residential preference during the pandemic.

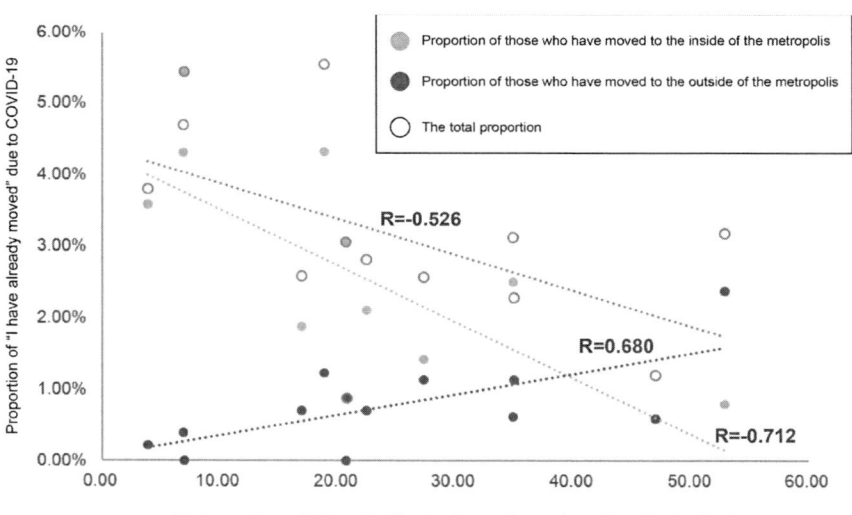

Fig. 5: Relationships between proportions of "I have already moved" and distance from Tokyo Station (Illustration: Keisuke Sakamoto, Marco Amati, Makoto Yokohari)

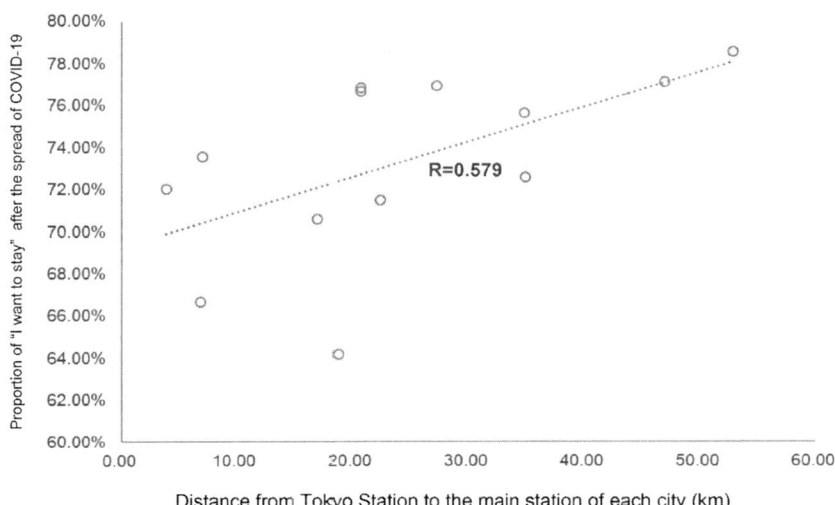

Fig. 6: Relationships between proportions of "I want to move" and distance from Tokyo Station (Illustration: Keisuke Sakamoto, Marco Amati, Makoto Yokohari)

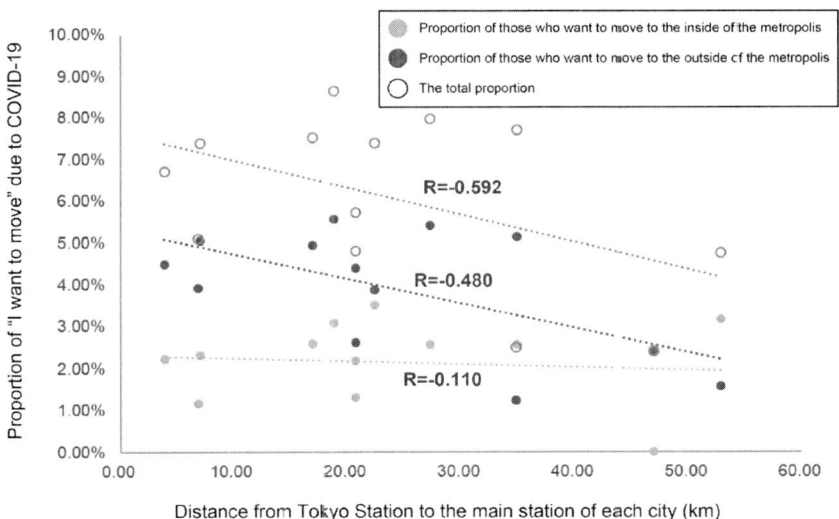

Fig. 7: Relationships between proportions of "I want to stay" and distance from Tokyo Station (Illustration: Keisuke Sakamoto, Marco Amati, Makoto Yokohari)

	Variables	Model 1 with only individual variables COEF (with 95 %CI)	
Threshold	„I want to move" | „I have no idea"	-2.86 (-3.00--2.72)	***
	„I have no idea" | „I have already moved" or „I want to stay"	-1.26 (-1.35--1.18)	***
Individual level factors	Sex	0.02 (-0.07-0.11)	
	Age	0.11 (0.01-0.21)	**
	Length of residency	-0.04 (-0.14-0.06)	
	Marital status	-0.01 (-0.12-0.09)	
	Number of family members	0.03 (-0.09-0.14)	
	Household income	0.08 (-0.01-0.17)	*
	Daily use of private car	-0.03 (-0.12-0.05)	
	(Ref. Owner-occupied detached house)	0.00	
	Owner-occupied flat	-0.08 (-0.19-0.03)	***
	Rental detached house	-0.14 (-0.21--0.07)	***
	Rental flat	-0.57 (-0.68--0.45)	***
	Public housing	-0.21 (-0.29--0.13)	***
	Company housing	-0.24 (-0.31--0.17)	***
	Shared house	-0.14 (-0.21--0.07)	***
	Other types of housing	-0.10 (-0.17--0.03)	***
	(Ref. Private company employee)	0.00	
	Public servant	0.00 (-0.08-0.09)	
	Self-employed	-0.04 (-0.13-0.04)	
	Freelance	-0.08 (-0.16-0.00)	**
	Temporary worker	0.02 (-0.07-0.11)	
	Part-time employee	0.03 (-0.07-0.13)	
	Change in teleworking frequency	-0.09 (-0.17-0.00)	**
	Commuting distance	-0.13 (-0.19--0.06)	***
Neighbourhood and municipality level factors	Population density		
	(Ref. Proportion of low residential land use)		
	Proportion of tall residential land use		
	Proportion of commercial land use		
	Proportion of industrial land use		
	Catchment area density of small park (250m radius)		
	Catchment area density of medium park (500m radius)		
	Catchment area density of large park (1,000m radius)		
	Catchment area density of multi-purpose park (1,000m radius)		
	Agricultural land density		
	Forest density		
	Distance from CBD		
	Land price		
	Day-night ratio of population in 2015		
	Change in day-night ratio of population from 1995 to 2015		
***P ≤ 0.01, **P ≤ 0.05, *P ≤ 0.1	N	3439	
	AIC	4529,6	

Table 3: Relationships between residential preference of three levels and socio-geographical factors

	Model 2 FULL model COEF (with 95%CI)		Model 3 optimised based on AIC COEF (with 95%CI)	
Threshold	-2.87 (-3.01--2.73)	***	-2.86 (-3.01--2.72)	***
	-1.27 (-1.35--1.18)	***	-1.26 (-1.35--1.18)	***
Individual level factors	0.02 (-0.07-0.11)			
	0.11 (0.01-0.21)	**	0.10 (0.01-0.18)	**
	-0.04 (-0.14-0.06)			
	-0.01 (-0.12-0.09)			
	0.03 (-0.09-0.14)			
	0.06 (-0.03-0.16)		0.06 (-0.02-0.14)	
	-0.02 (-0.11-0.08)			
	0.00		0.00	
	-0.12 (-0.24--0.01)	**	-0.10 (-0.21-0.01)	*
	-0.15 (-0.22--0.08)	***	-0.15 (-0.22--0.07)	***
	-0.60 (-0.72--0.48)	***	-0.57 (-0.67--0.48)	***
	-0.22 (-0.30--0.14)	***	-0.21 (-0.28--0.13)	***
	-0.25 (-0.32--0.18)	***	-0.24 (-0.31--0.17)	***
	-0.14 (-0.21--0.07)	***	-0.13 (-0.20--0.07)	***
	-0.11 (-0.18--0.04)	***	-0.10 (-0.17--0.03)	***
	0.00		0.00	
	0.00 (-0.09-0.08)			
	-0.04 (-0.13-0.04)			
	-0.08 (-0.16-0.00)	**	-0.09 (-0.16--0.01)	**
	0.02 (-0.07-0.11)			
	0.03 (-0.07-0.13)			
	-0.09 (-0.17-0.00)	**	-0.10 (-0.18--0.01)	**
	-0.13 (-0.19--0.06)	***	-0.12 (-0.18--0.05)	***
Neighbourhood and municipality level factors	0.06 (-0.09-0.22)			
	0.00			
	0.04 (-0.06-0.14)			
	0.03 (-0.08-0.13)			
	0.05 (-0.05-0.15)			
	-0.07 (-0.16-0.02)		-0.08 (-0.16-0.00)	**
	0.03 (-0.07-0.12)			
	-0.01 (-0.10-0.08)			
	0.03 (-0.06-0.12)			
	0.06 (-0.05-0.17)			
	-0.05 (-0.15-0.05)			
	0.12 (-0.02-0.27)	*	0.08 (-0.03-0.19)	
	0.16 (0.00-0.33)	*	0.17 (0.03-0.31)	**
	-0.01 (-0.14-0.12)			
	0.09 (-0.07-0.24)		0.08 (-0.02-0.19)	
***P ≤ 0.01, **P ≤ 0.05, *P ≤ 0.1	3439		3439	
	4541,6		4512,6	

Table 3: Relationships between residential preference of three levels and socio-geographical factors

Relations between residential preference and socio-geographical factors

At the beginning of analyses, DEFFs of between neighbourhoods or municipalities were calculated to decide whether single-level analyses or multilevel analyses should be utilised in the estimation of relationships between residential preferences and socio-geographical factors. The DEFFs of neighbourhood-level and municipality-level were 1.00 and 1.43, both of which are less than the standard value of 2.0, and hence the following analyses adopted single-level ordinal logistic regression models.

Table 3 shows the relationships between residential preference and socio-geographical factors through ordinal logistic regression analyses. The variance inflation factors (VIFs) of all the explanatory variables are less than 5.0, which indicates that there was no considerable multicollinearity between them. The results of Model 1 with only individual level factors indicate that age and household income have strong positive relations to the residential satisfaction, whereas people living either in an owner-occupied flat, a rental detached house, a rental flat, public housing, company housing, or a shared house all had a stronger negative relationship to residential satisfaction compared with those who are living in an owner-occupied detached house (the reference category of the eight housing types). As for conditions of employment and commuting, freelance workers have a stronger negative relation to the residential satisfaction compared to private company employees (the reference category of the six job types), and increasing teleworking frequency and commuting distance also negatively relates to residential satisfaction.

The results of Model 2 (FULL model) indicate comparatively strong positive relationships between the residential satisfaction and three neighbourhood and municipality level factors: distance to CBD from neighbourhoods, land prices of neighbourhoods, and change in day-night ratios of population from 1995 to 2015 of municipalities, while day-night ratio of population in 2015 has no significant relationship and its coefficient is negative. Relationships with other neighbourhood and municipality level factors are also insignificant, but it is notable that although the catchment area density of all types of parks has a negative or almost no relation with residential satisfaction, the density of agricultural land are positively related. Regarding individual level factors, their coefficients in Model 1 and Model 2 indicated almost the same relations.

Model 3 was optimised based on AIC and it indicates that among the neighbourhood and municipality level factors, distance from CBD, land price, and change in day-night ratio of population from 1995 to 2015 have significant relations with the residential preferences affected by the spread of COVID-19. In addition, catchment area density of small parks has also a significant negative relationship with the residential preferences.

Moreover, to identify heterogeneity of relations between various individuals and the neighbourhood and municipality level factors, interactions between individual level factors (age, household income, freelance worker, change in teleworking frequency, and commuting distance) and neighbourhood and municipality level factors (distance from CBD, land price, change in day-night ratio of population from 1995 to 2015) were examined on the basis of whether the AIC of Model 3 was improved or not by adding the interactions of the factors. Table 4 shows the coefficients of the interactions between the individual level factors and neighbourhood and municipality level factors in Model 3, and it expresses three significant relations; the more frequently people are able to telework after the spread of COVID-19, the greater the distance to which they are willing to relocate from central Tokyo; the older people are, the more willing they are to relocate to areas with high land price; and those who commute long distances prefer areas with a high day-night population ratio but seek lower land prices.

	Distance from CBD	Land price	Change in day-night ratio of population from 1995 to 2015
Age	-0.05 (-0.13–0.03)	**0.06 (-0.02–0.14)**	-0.05 (-0.13–0.03)
Household income	-0.03 (-0.10–0.05)	0.03 (-0.05–0.11)	0.00 (-0.07–0.08)
Freelance	0.01 (-0.07–0.08)	-0.04 (-0.12–0.04)	0.03 (-0.04–0.09)
Change in teleworking frequency	**0.10 (0.01–0.19)****	-0.05 (-0.13–0.04)	0.04 (-0.03–0.12)
Commuting distance	0.04 (-0.04–0.12)	**-0.06 (-0.14–0.02)**	**0.09 (-0.02–0.20)**
***P < 0.01, **P < 0.05, *P < 0.1 **Bold type:** models superior to Model 3 based on AIC			

Table 4: Coefficients of interaction between individual level factors and neighbourhood and city level factors added to Model 3

Distance from Tokyo Station	Number of neighbourhoods with estimated probability	Number of neighbourhoods with estimated probability of under 75 %	Proportion of neighbourhoods with estimated probability of under 75 %
D<15	1,693	176	10,40 %
15≤D<30	2,749	318	11,57 %
30≤D<45	2,907	444	15,27 %
45≤D	1,204	87	7,23 %

Table 5: Classification of estimated residential preferences of neighbourhoods according to the distance from Tokyo Station

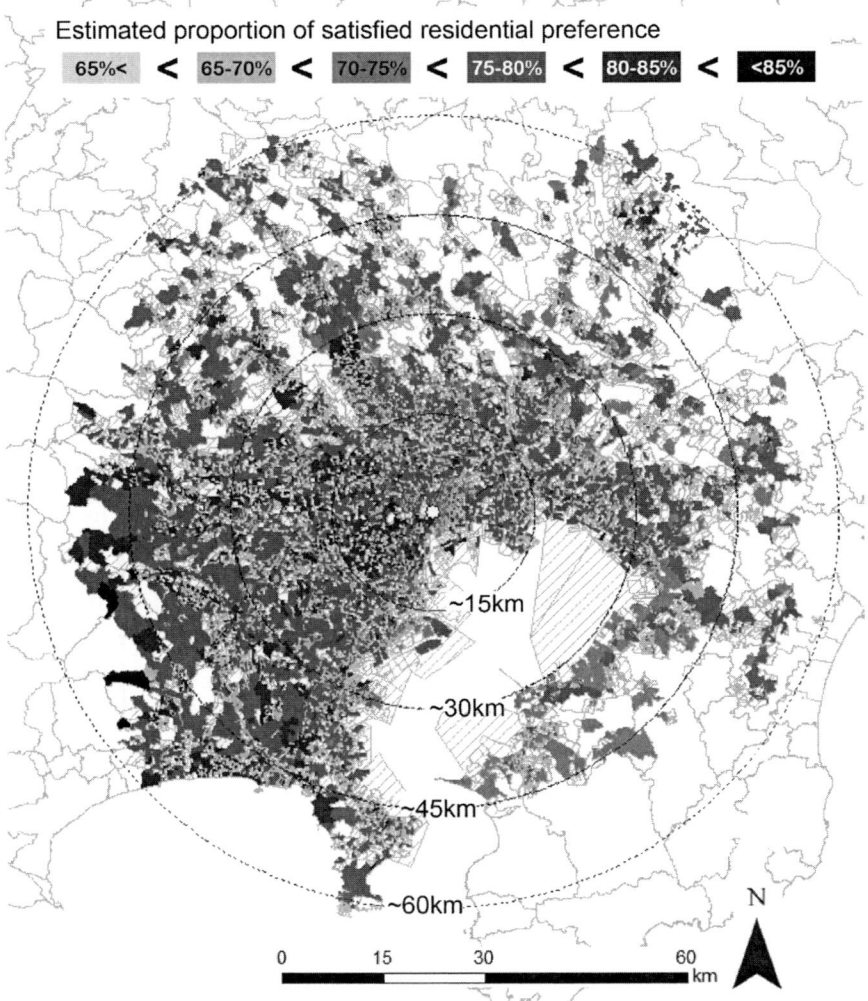

Fig. 8: Distribution of estimated residential preferences of the neighbourhoods in the Tokyo metropolitan area (Illustration: Keisuke Sakamoto, Marco Amati, Makoto Yokohari)

There are 8,553 neighbourhoods in the Tokyo metropolitan area including urban areas that have official data for all the neighbourhood and municipality level factors in Model 3. Residential preferences of an average person in the 8,553 neighbourhoods were then estimated based on the coefficients of Model 3, and the results of estimation were classified into four categories according to the distance from the Tokyo Station at every 15 kms (Table 5). Focusing on neighbourhoods with less than 75 % of estimated residential preference of "I have already moved" or "I want to stay" (c.f. the mean proportion of the questionnaire data: 76.13 %), the proportion of less satisfied neighbourhoods monotonically increases according to the distance from the Tokyo Station within the range of 45 km, but these unsatisfied neighbourhoods rapidly decreases between the range of 45 to 60 km, which suggests a possible tendency toward polarised residential preferences between the centre and outer suburbs due to the spread of COVID-19.

Interpretation of results

Theories of individual life course explain a diversity of relations between age and lifestyle such as residential location choice[1,2]. Prior to COVID-19 residential mobility was argued to depend on the life course[3,4,5]. Clark[5] identified through a case in Australia that the older people got above the age of 20, the less likely they were to move, and people living in owner-occupied housing were also less likely to move than those living in rental housing. In addition, van Ommeren et al.[7] argued that residential mobility was closely related to job mobility and commuting distance.

The results of the analyses about using individual factors seem consistent with that previous knowledge on residential mobility, suggesting that those who get to prefer to move after the pandemic are largely the young, able to use some discretion in arranging their working conditions like freelance workers, and those living in rental housing. Moreover, even for employees, if their offices are far from their residential neighbourhoods, they are also likely to have a preference for moving. One of the biggest changes between before and during the pandemic

---

[1] Elder, "Time, Human Agency, and Social Change: Perspectives on the Life Course."
[2] Wanberg et al., "Age and Reemployment Success After Job Loss: An Integrative Model and Meta-Analysis."
[3] Dieleman, "Modelling Residential Mobility: A Review of Recent Trends in Research. Journal of Housing and the Built Environment."
[4] Winstanley, Thorns and Perkins, "Moving House, Creating Home: Exporing Residential Mobility."
[5] Coulter, Ham and Findlay, "Re-Thinking Residential Mobility: Linking Lives Through Time and Space."
[6] Clark, "Life Course Events and Residential Change: Unpacking Age Effects on the Probability of Moving."
[7] Ommeren, "Job Mobility, Residential Mobility and Commuting: A Theoretical Analysis Using Search Theory."

is prevalence of teleworking, the frequency of which seems to have considerable impacts on residential mobility as implied in a study of Greece[8].

Upon controlling for the effects of the individual factors above, neighbourhood and municipality level factors' effects on residential preference seem to support the introduced hypothesis: residential location preference in a megacity after the pandemic has been polarised in a tug-of-war between the urban attraction for the centre of the metropolis and the attraction of natural amenities in the outer suburbs. The results suggest that two neighbourhood level factors, land prices of neighbourhoods as a proxy for access to urban jobs and services and distance from CBD as a proxy for access to natural amenities, are both positively related to residential satisfaction after the pandemic. In the study site, there is a negative correlation between the land price and distance, which fits with the line pre-COVID 19 in the hypothetical diagram of Fig. 1 and the shape of the left-hand side of the U-shaped line.

However, the latest day-night ratio of population, another proxy for urban attraction related to aggregation of daytime population, has no strong relations with the residential preference. Of the 13 study municipalities, Shibuya has by far the highest day-night ratio of population in 2015 (240.1%) and the second highest is Koto (122.2%). It could have been inferred that the urban amenity of these central wards contributes to the resilience of residential preference, but in fact, the overcrowding daytime populations might also have decreased the residential satisfaction of these areas during the pandemic.

Although the day-night ratio of population itself seems to have no significant influence on residential satisfaction, the prevailing increase in the day-night ratio of population before COVID-19 has a significant positive relationship. The change in day-night ratio of population indicates an inter-municipal change of population dynamics in the metropolitan area before COVID-19. To take examples in the study site, Musashino and Atsugi, some of the suburban cities with a comparatively highly dense commercial or business clusters[9], had been decreasing their ratio of day-night population from 1995 to 2015 (Musashino: 114.0% to 108.7%, Atsugi: 119.4% to 115.6%), while other suburban cities such as Tama or Kashiwa have experienced sharp increase (Tama: 82.6% to 101.0%, Kashiwa: 83.7% to 90.4%). These sharp increases among certain suburban cities reflect a competitive inter-municipal scramble for share of the daytime

---

[8] Mouratidis and Papagiannakis, "COVID-19, Internet, and Mobility: The Rise of Telework, Telehealth, E-Learning, and E-Shopping."
[9] Kumakoshi, Koizumi and Yoshimura, "Diversity and Density of Urban Functions in Station Areas."

population over the last two decades. Clearly this scramble will become more intense as the overall amount of the daytime population decreases as a result of residential preferences after the pandemic.

Future retrofit of inner suburbs with / after COVID-19

The argument that there is a polarisation of residential preference between the centre of the metropolis and outer suburbs in Tokyo, indicates that an increasing number of people will move to either of these areas after the COVID-19 pandemic subsides, whereas inner suburbs, most of which have been developed specifically as commuter towns without distinctive urban or natural features, are likely to face population decline, and especially an outflow of younger people. The results suggest that municipalities at the range of 30 to 45 km from Tokyo Station in particular need measures to prevent large population outflows.

Most inner suburban cities have relied on a connection to the centre of Tokyo for jobs and urban amenities, but the pandemic's lockdowns, teleworking and re-localisation of movement combined with an existing focus on the "15-Minute City" concept[10] mean that residents will continue to desire more accessible urban and natural attractions from their local neighbourhoods. A reallocation of infrastructural resources for re-equipping these areas for a post-pandemic future will have to focus on community building to build compatibility among residents of a neighbourhood and to form comfortable environments for teleworking[11].

It might be expected that natural and spacious attraction of inner suburbs are complemented by parks distributed all around cities, but the results of this study imply that proximity to small parks fails to mitigate the low residential satisfaction that people are likely to feel in these areas anyway. However, small parks, which are designed and arranged uniformly as ubiquitous spaces for recreation or relaxation which are free for residents to access, have the most negative influence. A reason may be that demand for urban green space has been diversifying and duplicated parks will not increase residential satisfaction[12]. Agricultural land, which indicates the strongest positive influence on the residential satisfaction of all the green land uses, could be re-evaluated as

---

[10] Guzman et.al., "COVID-19, Activity and Mobility Patterns in Bogotá. Are We Ready for a '15-Minute City'?"

[11] Carillo et al., "Adjusting to Epidemic-Induced Telework: Empirical Insights from Teleworkers in France."

[12] Kim et al., "Understanding Services from Ecosystem and Facilities Provided by Urban Green Spaces: A Use of Partial Profile Choice Experiment."

a key element to meet diverse demands for urban green space from various perspectives like improving thermal environment of neighbourhoods[13], providing productive activities for citizens[14], and raising biodiversity[15]. Furthermore, although the assumed depopulation after the pandemic in inner suburbs may accelerate the recent increase in the number of vacant lots,[16] conversion of vacant lots into urban agricultural spaces is one example in promoting of residents' preference for their neighbourhoods and cities[17]. Following Yokohari & Amati's[18] argument, the mixed pattern of agricultural and urban land use is a special feature of the geographical structure of Tokyo, and hence utilisation of existing urban agricultural land could optimise the amenity of inner suburban Tokyo through greenery and space as a guiding strategic principle for retrofitting during and after COVID-19.

Conclusion

The COVID-19 pandemic has had disruptive effect and will therefore lead to more unequal incomes, capital assets and wellbeing over time[19,20,21]. So far, this is the first study we know of that demonstrates how the pandemic has acted as a disruptive force to unsettle and redistribute established trends in housing preference across a megacity, with implications for land prices, infrastructure allocation and urban form. While land prices on the fringes of cities can curve upwards, replicating our hypothesised Figure 1, and clustering 'higher income groups trading off improved environmental consumption over increased journey times'[22], this trend

---

[13] Yokohari et al., "Effects of Paddy Fields on Sum-Mertime Air and Surface Temperatures in Urban Fringe Areas of Tokyo, Japan."
[14] Dunlap, Harmon and Kyle, "Growing in Place: The Interplay of Urban Agriculture and Place Sentiment."
[15] Lin, Philpott and Jha, "The Future of Urban Agriculture and Biodiversity-Ecosystem Services.: Challenges and Next Steps."
[16] Usui and Perez, "Are Patterns of Vacant Lots Random? Evidence from Empirical Spatiotemporal Analysis in Chiba Prefecture, East of Tokyo."
[17] Tong et al., "Optimize Urban Food Production to Address Food Deserts in Regions with Restricted Water Access."
[18] Yokohari and Amati, "Nature in the City, City in the Nature: Case Studies of the Resto-Ration of Urban Nature in Tokyo, Japan and Toronto, Canada."
[19] Oronce et al., "Association Between State-Level Income Inequality and COVID-19 Cases and Mortality in the USA."
[20] Berrera-Algarín et al., "COVID-19, neoliberalismo y sistemas sanitarios en 30 países de Europa: repercusiones en el número de fallecidos."
[21] Tatar et al., "International COVID-19 Vaccine Inequality Amid the Pandemic: Perpetuating a Global Crisis?"
[22] McCann, *The UK Regional-National Economic Problem: Geography, Globalisation and Governance*, 326.

is usually attributed to schemes that preserve these areas such as a greenbelt and not to the effects of a pandemic.

At the same time, at the megalopolitan level, a polarizing effect on the metropolitan area caused by an epi- or pandemic is not without historical precedent. London, as one of the earliest and most globally connected megacities saw the birth of suburban living during the 17th to 19th centuries in successive waves, due in part to a 'form follows fear of infection model'[23] but also through great wealth, since travel, although frequent by 'short stage' coaches, was well beyond the means of ordinary individuals[24]. Not only were these individuals motivated by a desire for natural beauty but also by a misplaced fear that diseases, such as cholera, were transmitted by stagnant low-lying air[25,26]. Similar to the epidemics of the 19th century, the impact of 'urban long-COVID' is likely to be multi-generational. For example, the effect of the 1854 cholera epidemic on house prices in London persisted for 160 years[27].

This study has focused on a contemporary megacity and demonstrated that disease as a driver of suburbanisation remains current in the 21st century, using an online questionnaire survey and ordinal logistic regression analyses on the relationships between residential preference and socio-geographical factors. We have discussed the implications of these findings and how they are likely to affect the future retrofit of inner suburbs that already face long term population decline.

Although the results of this study showed relationships between residential preference and socio-geographical factors at one point of the pandemic, a remaining unknown and gap for future enquiry is how path dependent these relationships are into the future even after the pandemic subsides. In addition, how residential preference will drive actual behaviour in selecting or changing residential location is also unknown, and therefore, continuous surveys on associations between residential preference and residential mobility are required. Furthermore, people younger than 40 years old called as "Millennials" and "Generation Z"

---

[23] Megahed and Ghoneim, "Antivirus-Built Environment: Lessons Learned from Covid-19 Pandemic."
[24] Besant, *History of London*, 214.
[25] Amati, *The City and the Super-Organism: A History of Naturalism in Urban Planning*, 46.
[26] White, *London in the 19th Century: A Human Awful Wonder of God*, 88.
[27] Ambrus, Field and Gonzalez. "Loss in the Time of Cholera: Long-Run Impact of a Disease Epidemic on the Urban Landscape."

are known to have distinct sense of values from older generations[28,29,30,31]. Such generational attitudes must also be considered when considering or arguing for a long-term shift in residential preference before and after COVID-19.

Bibliography

Amati, Marco. *The City and the Super-Organism: A History of Naturalism in Urban Planning.* Singapore: Palgrave Macmillan, 2021.

Ambrus, Attila, Erica Field, and Robert Gonzalez. "Loss in the Time of Cholera: Long-Run Impact of a Disease Epidemic on the Urban Landscape." *The American economic review*, 2020. https://doi.org/10.1257/aer.20190759.

Asakawa, Tatsuto. "Changes in the Socio-Spatial Structure in the Tokyo Metropolitan Area: Social Area Analysis of Changes from 1990 to 2010." *Develpoment and Society* 45, no. 3 (2016): 537–62.

Barrera-Algarín, Evaristo, Francisco Estepa-Maestre, José Luís Sarasola-Sánchez-Serrano, and Ana Vallejo-Andrada. "COVID-19, neoliberalismo y sistemas sanitarios en 30 países de Europa: repercusiones en el número de fallecidos." *Revista espanola de salud publica* 94 (2020).

Besant, Walter. *History of London.* London: Longmans, Green and Co, 1894.

Carillo, Kevin, Gaëlle Cachat-Rosset, Josianne Marsen, Tania Saba, and Alain Klarsfeld. "Adjusting to Epidemic-Induced Telework: Empirical Insights from Teleworkers in France." *European Journal of information systems* 2021, no. 30 (1): 69–88.

Champion, Anthony G. G. "Urban and Regional Demographic Trends in the Developed World." *Urban Studies*, no. 29 (1992): 461–82.

Clark, William A. V. "Life Course Events and Residential Change: Unpacking Age Effects on the Probability of Moving." *Journal of Population Research*, 2013, 319–34.

Coulter, Rory, Maarten van Ham, and Allan M. Findlay. "Re-Thinking Residential Mobility: Linking Lives Through Time and Space." *Progress in human geography* 40, no. 3 (2016): 352–74. https://doi.org/10.1177/0309132515575417.

Da Schio, Nicola, Amy Phillips, Koos Fransen, Manuel Wolff, Dagmar Haase, Silvija Krajter Ostoić, and Ivana Živojinović et al. "The Impact of the COVID-19 Pandemic on the Use of and Attitudes Towards Urban Forests and Green Spaces: Exploring the Instigators of Change in Belgium." *Urban Forestry & Urban Greening* 65 (2021): 127305. https://doi.org/10.1016/j.ufug.2021.127305.

---

[28] McDonald, "Are Millennials Really the "Go-Nowhere" Generation?"
[29] Lee, "Are Millennials Coming to Town? Residential Location Choice of Young Adults."
[30] Ehlenz, Pfeiffer and Pearthree, "Downtown Revitalization in the Era of Millennials: How Developer Perceptions of Millennial Market Demands Are Shaping Urban Landscapes."
[31] Giachino et al., "Urban Area and Nature-Based Solution: Is This an Attractive Solution for Generation Z?"

Devine-Wright, Patrick, Laís Pinto de Carvalho, Andrés Di Masso, Maria Lewicka, Lynne Manzo, and Daniel R. Williams. "'Re-Placed'- Reconsidering Relationships with Place and Lessons from a Pandemic." *Journal of Environmental Psychology* 72 (2020). https://doi.org/10.1016/j.jenvp.2020.101514.

Dieleman, Frans M. "Modelling Residential Mobility: A Review of Recent Trends in Research. Journal of Housing and the Built Environment." *Journal of Housing and the Built Environment*, no. 16 (2001): 249–65.

Douglas, Margaret, Srinivasa Vittal Katikireddi, Martin Taulbut, Martin McKee, and Gerry McCartney. "Mitigating the Wider Health Effects of Covid-19 Pandemic Response." *BMJ*, 2020, m1557. https://doi.org/10.1136/bmj.m1557.

Dunlap, Rudy, Justin Harmon, and Gerard Kyle. "Growing in Place: The Interplay of Urban Agriculture and Place Sentiment." *Leisure/Loisir* 37, no. 4 (2013): 397–414. https://doi.org/10.1080/14927713.2014.906173.

Ehlenz, Meagan M., Deirdre Pfeiffer, and Genevieve Pearthree. "Downtown Revitalization in the Era of Millennials: How Developer Perceptions of Millennial Market Demands Are Shaping Urban Landscapes." *Urban Geography* 41, no. 1 (2020): 79–102. https://doi.org/10.1080/02723638.2019.1647062.

Elder, Glen H. Jr. "Time, Human Agency, and Social Change: Perspectives on the Life Course." *Social Psychology Quarterly* Quarterly (1994): 4–15.

Finucane, Melissa L., Robin Beckman, Madhumita Gosh-Dastidar, Tamara Dubowitz, Rebecca L. Collins, and Wendy Troxel. "Do Social Isolation and Neighbourhood Walkability Influence Relationships Between COVID-19 Experiences and Wellbeing in Predominantly Black Urban Areas?" *Landscape and Urban Planning*, no. 217 (2022). https://doi.org/10.1016/j.landurbplan.2021.104264.

Fishman, Robert. "Longer View: The Fifth Migration." *Journal of the American Planning Association* 71, no. 4 (2005): 357–66.

Foley, Donald L. "Urban Daytime Population: A Field for Demographic-Ecological Analysis." *Social Forces* 32, no. 4 (1954): 323–30.

Giachino, Chiara, Luigi Bollani, Elisa Truant, and Alessandro Boradonna. "Urban Area and Nature-Based Solution: Is This an Attractive Solution for Generation Z?" *Land Use Policy* 112 (2022). https://doi.org/10.1016/j.landusepol.2021.105828.

Gür, Miray. "Post-Pandemic Lifestyle Changes and Their Interaction with Resident Behavior in Housing and Neighborhoods: Bursa, Turkey." *Journal of Housing and the Built Environment* 37, no. 2 (2022): 823–62. https://doi.org/10.1007/s10901-021-09897-y.

Guzman, Luis A., Julián Arellna, Daniel Oviedo Oviedo, and Carlos Alberto Moncada Aristizábal. "COVID-19, Activity and Mobility Patterns in Bogotá. Are We Ready for a '15-Minute City'?" *Travel Behaviour and Society*, no. 24 (2021): 245–56.

Haas, Mathijs de, Roel Faber, and Marije Hamersma. "How COVID-19 and the Dutch 'Intelligent Lockdown' Change Activities, Work and Travel Behaviour: Evidence from Longitudinal Data in the Netherlands." *Transportation Research Interdisciplinary Perspectives* 6 (2020). https://doi.org/10.1016/j.trip.2020.100150.

Hall, Peter Geoffrey. *Cities in Civilization*. London: Phoenix Giant, 1998.

Hyra, Derek. "The Back-to-the-City Movement: Neighbourhood Redevelopment and Processes of Political and Cultural Displacement." *Urban Studies* 52, no. 10 (2015): 1753–73.

Jones, Antwan, and Diana S. Grigsby-Toussaint. "Housing Stability and the Residential Context of the COVID-19 Pandemic." *Cities & Health* 5 (2021): 159-S161. https://doi.org/10.1080/23748834.2020.1785164.

Kim, Hyerin, Yasushi Shoji, Takahiro Tsuge, Tetsuya Aikoh, and Koichi Kuriyama. "Understanding Services from Ecosystem and Facilities Provided by Urban Green Spaces: A Use of Partial Profile Choice Experiment." *Forest Policy and Economics* 111 (2020). https://doi.org/10.1016/j.forpol.2019.102086.

Kumakoshi, Yusuke, Hideki Koizumi, and Yuji Yoshimura. "Diversity and Density of Urban Functions in Station Areas." *Computers, Environment and Urban Systems* 89 (2021). https://doi.org/10.1016/j.compenvurbsys.2021.101679.

Lee, Hyojung. "Are Millennials Coming to Town? Residential Location Choice of Young Adults." *Urban Affairs Review* 56, no. 2 (2020): 565–604.

Lees, Loretta. "Gentrification and Social Mixing: Towards an Inclusive Urban Renaissance?" *Urban Studies* 45, no. 12 (2008): 2249–2470.

Lehberger, Mira, Anne-Katrin Kleih, and Kai Sparke. "Self-Reported Well-Being and the Importance of Green Spaces – a Comparison of Garden Owners and Non-Garden Owners in Times of COVID-19." *Landscape and Urban Planning* 212 (2021). https://doi.org/10.1016/j.landurbplan.2021.104108.

Lin, Breanda B., Stacy M. Philpott, and Shalena Jha. "The Future of Urban Agriculture and Biodiversity-Ecosystem Services.: Challenges and Next Steps." *Basic and Applied Ecology*, no. 16 (2021): 189–201. https://doi.org/10.1016/j.baae.2015.01.005.

McCann, Philip. *The UK Regional-National Economic Problem: Geography, Globalisation and Governance*. Regions and Cities. London: Routledge, 2016.

McDonald, Noreen C. "Are Millennials Really the "Go-Nowhere" Generation?" *Journal of the American Planning Association* 81, no. 2 (2015): 90–103. https://doi.org/10.1080/01944363.2015.1057196.

Megahed, Naglaa A., and Ehab M. Ghoneim. "Antivirus-Built Environment: Lessons Learned from Covid-19 Pandemic." *Sustainable Cities and Society* 61 (2020). https://doi.org/10.1016/j.scs.2020.102350.

Mieszkowski, Peter, and Edwin Smith Mills. "The Causes of Metropolitan Suburbanization." *Journal of Economic Perspectives* 7, no. 3 (1993): 135–47.

Mouratidis, Kostas. "How COVID-19 Reshaped Quality of Life in Cities: A Synthesis and Implications for Urban Planning." *Land Use Policy* 111 (2021). https://doi.org/10.1016/j.landusepol.2021.105772.

Mouratidis, Kostas, and Apostolos Papagiannakis. "COVID-19, Internet, and Mobility: The Rise of Telework, Telehealth, E-Learning, and E-Shopping." *Sustainable Cities and Society* 74 (2021). https://doi.org/10.1016/j.scs.2021.103182.

Muthen, Bengt O., and Albert Satorra. "Complex Sample Data in Structural Equation Modeling." *Sociological methodology* 25 (1995): 267-316.

Ohashi, Hiroaki, and Nicholas A. Phelps. "Diversity in Decline: The Changing Suburban Fortunes of Tokyo Metropolis." *Cities*, no. 103 (2020). https://doi.org/10.1016/j.cities.2020.102693.

Ohashi, Hiroaki, and Nicholas A. Phelps. "Contrasts in Suburban Decline: A Tale of Three Key Outer Suburban 'Business Core Cities' in Tokyo Metropolis." *Urban Geography* 44, no. 1 (2023): 149-77. https://doi.org/10.1080/02723638.2021.1963556.

Oishi, Shigehiro, Youngjae Cha, and Ulrich Schimmack. "The Social Ecology of COVID-19 Cases and Deaths in New York City: The Role of Walkability, Wealth, and Race." *Social Psychological and Person-ality Science* 12, no. 8 (2021): 1457-66.

Ommeren, Jos van, Piet Rietveld, and Peter Nijkamp. "Job Mobility, Residential Mobility and Commuting: A Theoretical Analysis Using Search Theory." *The Annals of Regional Science* 34 (2000): 213-32.

Oronce, Carlos Irwin A., Christopher A. Scannell, Ichiro Kawachi, and Yusuke Tsugawa. "Association Between State-Level Income Inequality and COVID-19 Cases and Mortality in the USA." *Journal of general internal medicine* 35, no. 9 (2020): 2791-93. https://doi.org/10.1007/s11606-020-05971-3.

Pagani, Anna, Livia Fritz, Ralph Hansmann, Vincent Kaufmann, and Claudia R. Binder. "How the First Wave of COVID-19 in Switzerland Affected Residential Preferences." *Cities & Health*, 2021, 1-13. https://doi.org/10.1080/23748834.2021.1982231.

Phelps, Nicholas A., and Hiroaki Ohashi. "Edge City Denied? The Rise and Fall of Tokyo's Outer Sub-Urban 'Business Core Cities'." *Journal of Planning Education and Research* 40, no. 4 (2018): 379-92.

Phelps, Nicholas A., David C. Valler, and Andrew M. Wood. "A Postsuburban World? An Outline of a Re-Search Agenda." *Environment and Planning A* 42, no. 2 (2010): 366-83.

Poortinga, Wouter, Natasha Bird, Britt Hallingberg, Rhiannon Phillips, and Denitza Williams. "The Role of Perceived Public and Private Green Space in Subjective Health and Wellbeing During and After the First Peak of the COVID-19 Outbreak." *Landscape and Urban Planning* 211 (2021). https://doi.org/10.1016/j.landurbplan.2021.104092.

Schulz, Evelyn. "Trends of Revitalizing Central City Peripheries in Tokyo." *disP - The Planning Review* 46, no. 181 (2010): 32-35.

Shakibaei, Shahin, Gerard C. de Jong, Pelin Alpkökin, and Taha H. Rashidi. "Impact of the COVID-19 Pandemic on Travel Behavior in Istanbul: A Panel Data Analysis." *Sustainable Cities and Society* 65 (2021). https://doi.org/10.1016/j.scs.2020.102619.

Shamshiripour, Ali, Ehsan Rahimi, Ramin Shabanpour, and Abolfazl Kouros Mohammadian. "How Is COVID-19 Reshaping Activity-Travel Behavior? Evidence from a Comprehensive Survey in Chicago." *Transportation Research Interdisciplinary Perspectives* 7 (2020). https://doi.org/10.1016/j.trip.2020.100216.

Sorensen, André. "Subcentres and Satellite Cities: Tokyo's 20th Century Experience of Planned Polycentrism." *International Planning Studies* 6, no. 1 (2001): 9–32. https://doi.org/10.1080/13563470120026505.

Sturtevant, Lisa A., and Ju Yin Jung. "Are We Moving Back to the City? Examining Residential Mobility in the Washington, DC Metropolitan Area." *Growth and Change* 42, no. 1 (2011): 48–91.

Sweeney, Glennon, and Bernadette Hanlon. "From Old Suburb to Post-Suburb: The Politics of Retrofit in the Inner Suburb of Upper Arlington, Ohio." *Journal of Urban Affairs*, no. 39 (2016): 241–59.

Tatar, Moosa, Jalal Montazeri Shoorekchali, Mohammad Reza Faraji, and Fernando A. Wilson. "International COVID-19 Vaccine Inequality Amid the Pandemic: Perpetuating a Global Crisis?" *Journal of global health* 11 (2021). https://doi.org/10.7189/jogh.11.03086.

Teixeira, João Filipe, and Miguel Lopes. "The Link Between Bike Sharing and Subway Use During the COVID-19 Pandemic: The Case-Study of New York's Citi Bike." *Transportation Research Interdisciplinary Perspectives* 6 (2020). https://doi.org/10.1016/j.trip.2020.100166.

Tong, Daoqin, Courtney Crosson, Qing Zhong, and Yinan Zhang. "Optimize Urban Food Production to Address Food Deserts in Regions with Restricted Water Access." *Landscape and Urban Planning* 202 (2020). https://doi.org/10.1016/j.landurbplan.2020.103859.

Ugolini, Francesca, Luciano Massetti, Pedro Calaza-Martínez, Paloma Cariñanos, Cynnamon Dobbs, Silvija Krajter Ostoić, and Ana Marija Marin et al. "Effects of the COVID-19 Pandemic on the Use and Perceptions of Urban Green Space: An International Exploratory Study." *Urban Forestry & Urban Greening* 56 (2020). https://doi.org/10.1016/j.ufug.2020.126888.

Usui, Hiroyuki, and Joan Perez. "Are Patterns of Vacant Lots Random? Evidence from Empirical Spatiotemporal Analysis in Chiba Prefecture, East of Tokyo." *Urban Analytics and City Science,* 1–17.

Wanberg, Connie R., Ruth Kanfer, Darla J. Hamann, and Zhen Zhang. "Age and Reemployment Success After Job Loss: An Integrative Model and Meta-Analysis." *Psychological Bulletin* 142, no. 4 (2016): 400–426. https://doi.org/10.1037/bul0000019.

White, Jerry. *London in the 19th Century: A Human Awful Wonder of God.* London: Vintage Books, 2007.

Winstanley, Ann, David C. Thorns, and Harvey C. Perkins. "Moving House, Creating Home: Exporing Residential Mobility." *Housing Studies* 17, no. 6 (2002): 813–32. https://doi.org/10.1080/02673030216000.

Yokohari, Makoto, and Marco Amati. "Nature in the City, City in the Nature: Case Studies of the Resto-Ration of Urban Nature in Tokyo, Japan and Toronto, Canada." *Landscape and Ecological Engineering* 1 (2005): 53–59.

Yokohari, Makoto, Robert D, Brown, Yoshitake Kato, and Hideki Moriyama. "Effects of Paddy Fields on Sum-Mertime Air and Surface Temperatures in Urban Fringe Areas of Tokyo, Japan." *Landscape and Urban Planning* 38 (1997): 1–11.

Zarrabi, Mahsa, Seyed-Abbas Yazdanfar, and Seyed-Bagher Hosseini. "COVID-19 and Healthy Home Preferences: The Case of Apartment Residents in Tehran." *Journal of Building Engineering* 35 (2021): 102021. https://doi.org/10.1016/j.jobe.2020.102021.

Chapter 2:
Transformation of Public Space

The Streets of Vienna in Times of the COVID-19 Pandemic – Transformation Processes of Public Space Through Walking, Cycling and Scootering

Irene Bittner

Introduction

As in many metropolises at the beginning of 2020, measures to contain the COVID-19 pandemic were put into place in Vienna leading to changes in mobility and the use of public space. Physical social contact was severely restricted – albeit temporarily – by the so-called "lockdowns". Daily travel was reduced to an absolute minimum. The technical possibilities of digitalisation led to many professionals working from home and educational activities taking place via distance learning. The use of video conferencing tools quickly became the norm for both work and education. As such, Vienna's streets suddenly became empty, especially during the first lockdowns, with hardly any cars driving through the city and public transport timetables being thinned out due to the dramatic drop in demand.

Walking, cycling and scootering gained more importance for mobility, exercise and recreation in one's own neighbourhood as people's freedom of movement was restricted and people began working from home. This resulted in sharply declining passenger numbers in public transport due to the very substantial reduction in people commuting to work and the obligation to wear a protective mask, which put many people off from using public transport. In turn this has led to a new boost in active mobility since March 2020.

This change has increased the pressure on public spaces such as streets, sidewalks, cycle paths, squares and parks. For example, the share of cycling in Vienna, seven percent in 2019, jumped to almost ten percent in 2020 increasing significantly more than in the last 20 years of the City of Vienna's active cycling policy.

Within the context of a climate-friendly transport transition, this article looks at the opportunities and challenges of the changes brought about by the COVID-19 pandemic, which have resulted in a switch to a more active mobility, as well as to a corresponding redesign of some streets and public spaces in Vienna. To this end, this contribution follows the thesis that the everyday practices which have changed due to responses to the pandemic rely on a broader political as well as social understanding and can contribute to (1) bringing the ratio of space consumption in car-friendly cities such as Vienna back into a better balance and (2) the demand for more public space for active transport, physical activities, interaction and for simply spending time in.

Uneven distribution of usable public space in Vienna

Public space and space for active transport are scarce commodities in Vienna – as indeed they are in many European cities. Urban research is therefore increasingly discussing the question of spatial or territorial justice for a wider variety of usage when it comes to the transformation of public space.[1,2,3] This concerns questions that focus on both physical-material and social space and, in recent times, has been increasingly focused on the consequences of the climate crisis such as the urban heat island effect. On the physical-material level, in the sense of a built urban environment, urban research deals with the questions of how urban space is designed and equipped or how urban space is conceived in planning terms. At the socio-spatial level, questions are pursued that deal with socio-economic and cultural practice and differentiated ways of using urban spaces.

An inequitable physical-material distribution related to everyday mobility in Vienna can be seen in the many narrow pavements in Vienna, where the recommended minimum width for pedestrians of two metres is not met:[4,5] According to a study by the Vienna University of Technology in the 1th to the 9th districts (the inner city districts), as well as in the 20th district between 16 to 27 percent of the pavements are less than two metres wide.[6] In the 11th to the 19th districts – which have densely built-up urban neighbourhoods closer to the city center and loosely built-up neighbourhoods on the outskirts of the city – about 24 to 55 percent of the pavements are less than two metres wide. In the

---

[1] Degros and Schwab, *Territorial Justice*.
[2] Fainstein, *The Just City*.
[3] Harvey, *Social Justice and the City – revised*.
[4] Österreichische Forschungsgesellschaft Straße – Schiene – Verkehr, "Fußgängerverkehr. Richtlinien und Vorschriften für das Straßenwesen – RVS 03.02.12."
[5] Brezina, Leth and Graser, "Pavement width Maps – District Comparison."
[6] Ibid.

more suburban 21th to 23rd districts about 42 to 62 percent of the pavements do not comply with the Austrian guidelines for pedestrian traffic and are also less than two metres wide.

In addition, most of Vienna's street spaces are primarily oriented to the needs of motorised traffic. In most streets, much more space is given to moving vehicles and to cars parked at the roadside than to active mobility such as walking, cycling and scootering. This is also illustrated by a study of the University of Natural Resources and Life Sciences, Vienna.[7] Compared to the cities of Copenhagen, Rotterdam, Barcelona and Munich, Vienna's side streets in densely built-up residential areas are at the bottom of the list with only 30 percent of space for active mobility. Similar streets in Copenhagen or Rotterdam have more than 45 percent.

Even before the COVID-19 pandemic, some streets in Vienna were being slowly but steadily converted into traffic-calmed zones, pedestrian zones (almost) without motor vehicle traffic or into encounter zones that do not require pavements and have a maximum speed limit of 20 kilometres per hour. A prominent example is the conversion of Mariahilfer Straße – one of Vienna's most important shopping streets – into a combined encounter zone and pedestrian zone, which took place during 2015. In the years that followed, car-free and traffic-calmed zones also followed in the surrounding streets and squares in the immediate vicinity of Mariahilfer Straße, such as Neubaugasse, Zollergasse or Otto-Bauer-Gasse.

Bicycle lanes and cycling infrastructure are increasingly being developed in each of Vienna's 23 districts. Decentralised planning competencies, however, means that the quality varies greatly from district to district. The implementation of cycling streets in Vienna began after their introduction into the Austrian Road Traffic Regulations Act (StVO) of 2013. Since 2019, there has been a master plan in place for cycling streets.[8] Canovagasse between The Ring and Karlsplatz in the centre of Vienna, and Goldschlaggasse and Hasnerstraße to the west were converted first with others following in 2020, coincidentally just in time for the start of the COVID-19 pandemic.

Regarding the socio-spatial level, i.e. in relation to the possibilities of using urban spaces, the reconstruction of the street and path network in favour of walking, cycling, scootering or simply spending time there is progressing rather

---

[7] Furchtlehner and Lička, "Back on the Street: Vienna, Copenhagen, Munich, and Rotterdam in focus."
[8] City of Vienna, Municipal Department 18 – Urban Development and Planning, "Masterplan Fahrradstraßen."

slowly in Vienna. An analysis of the University of Natural Resources and Life Sciences, Vienna, related to the socially just distribution of green spaces in Vienna states that there is an average of 9.26 m2 of parks per inhabitant compared to an area of 12.44 m2 for motorised traffic – minus the pavement areas and areas of structurally separated cycle paths.[9] The Danish capital Copenhagen, on the other hand, has been focusing on a largely car-free city centre and a corresponding design of public spaces since the 1990s. Since 2003, the French capital Paris has been working on significantly reducing the number of car parking spaces in public urban spaces and implementing a generous cycling infrastructure. Compared to other European cities, Vienna is rather hesitant in this regard, even though the pressure on Vienna's public space is particularly high in densely built-up residential areas and also makes redesigns such as climate crisis adaptation measures urgently necessary. This was specifically evident in 2020 and 2021, where the residential population of the inner-city districts in particular was dependent on nearby outdoor recreational space while people were working from home and engaged in distance learning.[10,11]

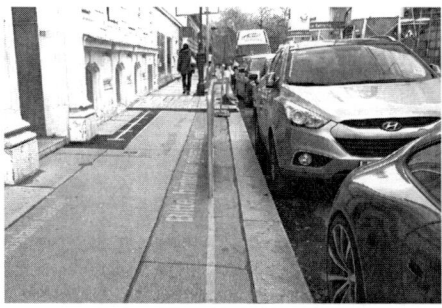 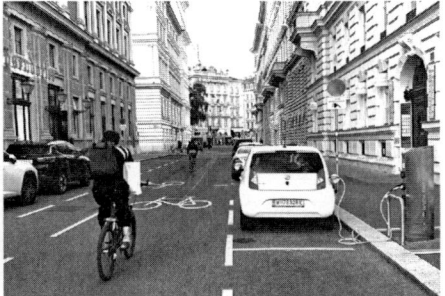

Fig. 1: COVID-19 distance marking on the narrow pavement in front of a school, 2022 (Photo: Irene Bittner)

Fig. 2: A new cycling street in Canovagasse, 2021 (Photo: Irene Bittner)

In the outer districts and suburbs of Vienna with a somewhat looser density of buildings and larger green areas available for nearby recreation, public spaces such as streets and squares are strongly oriented towards the needs of

---

[9] Reinwald et al., "Urban Green Infrastructure and Green Open Spaces: An Issue of Social Fairness in Times of COVID-19 Crisis."
[10] Ibid.
[11] Lehner et al., "Greenspace Justice in Vienna: A Research through Design Approach."

motorised traffic. In addition, shopping facilities and social infrastructure in suburban residential areas are organised on a larger scale and therefore often favour arrival by car. Longer distances and a lack of cycling and walking infrastructure in front of local shops, schools, kindergartens and health care facilities make work, supply, drop-off and pick-up trips by car the preferred choice.

Changes to the streets of Vienna brought about by the COVID-19 emergency and the lockdowns

At the beginning of 2020, the rapid spread of the SARS-CoV-2 virus created a global health situation that required repressive measures to contain the viral disease. Regulations such as lockdowns and the wearing of mouth-nose protection and later on FFP2-masks became the "new normal" and meant massive restrictions on social, economic and cultural life, especially for differentiated urban societies – as was the case in Vienna.

In Austria, and thus also in the federal capital Vienna, the first lockdown was declared on 16 March 2020, which resulted in the extensive closures of schools, kindergartens, universities and other educational institutions, restaurants, hotels and large parts of the retail sector, as well as the closure of sports and cultural venues such as cinemas, concert halls, theatres, fitness clubs, football pitches, indoor pools, museums and clubs.[12] People had to stay home, as curfews were also imposed. Leaving one's "own private living quarters" was only allowed under the following conditions: *"1. averting an immediate danger to life, limb and property, 2. caring for and helping persons in need of support as well as exercising family rights and fulfilling family duties, 3. meeting the necessary basic needs of daily life, 4. professional purposes, if this is necessary, and 5. spending time outdoors for physical and mental recreation."*[13] This first lockdown ended on 30 April 2020 but the opening of schools and the lifting of remaining restrictions on trade, gastronomy, culture and other facilities did not take place until 1 July 2020. Due to dramatic increases in the number of cases as the virus spread in waves and the appearance of new variants, further lockdowns were imposed in Austria on a stop-start basis and with regional variations up until the end of 2021.

In Vienna, people were particularly affected by the curfews during the lockdowns because a sufficient supply of urban spaces where people could spend time outdoors proved to be problematic in terms of spatial justice. An

---

[12] Pollak, Kowarz and Partheymüller, "Chronologie zur Corona-Krise in Österreich – Teil 1: Vorgeschichte, der Weg in den Lockdown, die akute Phase und wirtschaftliche Folgen."

[13] BGBl. I, "COVID-19 Maßnahmengesetz."

evaluation of the Austria-wide Corona Panel survey from April 2020 showed that predominantly the urban population – especially those with small flats under 35 m2 – do not have private open spaces such as a garden or balcony of their own. In Vienna, 27 percent of the population stated that they had no access to private green and open spaces. In inner-city areas, many people depended on a correspondingly small-scale distribution of public open spaces in their living environment. The narrow pavements in Vienna were often the only places where people could be outdoors and yet also close to home. According to the COVID-19 Measures Act from 2020, a distance of first two and later one metre had to be kept from other people who did not live in the same household.[14] As it was not clear at the time how infectious the Sars-CoV-2 virus was during physical contact outdoors, playgrounds in Vienna's parks and squares were temporarily closed during the first lockdown.[15] Also, parks managed by the federal government rather than the City of Vienna (e.g. Augarten Park in the inner city) remained closed, thereby denying thousands of people living in the vicinity access to valuable green spaces in the otherwise densely built-up urban area.[16] Only after intensive public discussions were these parks reopened on 14 April 2020 for "spending time outdoors for physical and mental recreation".

Especially during the first lockdown from 16 March to 30 April 2020, images of empty public spaces emerged.[17] Motorised traffic declined almost completely with active mobility such as walking and cycling also declining sharply in the first weeks.[18] In addition to the closures and exit restrictions, there were worldwide travel restrictions. Having a particular impact on Austria and Vienna, were the restrictions on freedom of travel within the European Union and the closure of borders between EU states that had been open for decades. This also greatly reduced long-distance mobility by train, bus or plane.[19] For Vienna as a popular destination for city tourism, as well as an internationally oriented conference, science, culture and trade city, not only important economic sources of revenue were lost, but also the otherwise busy public spaces in the city centre, which had previously been considered examples of overtourism, were largely deserted during this period.[20]

---

[14] Ibid.
[15] Ibid.
[16] Ibid.
[17] La Speranza, *Wien im Lockdown. Zwischen Stillstand und Hoffnung.*
[18] Hartwig et al., "The Impacts of a COVID-19 Related Lockdown (and Reopening Phases) on Time Use and Mobility for Activities in Austria-Results from a Multi-Wave Combined Survey."
[19] Jiricka-Pürrer, Brandenburg and Pröbstl-Haider, "City tourism pre- and post-covid-19 pandemic – Messages to take home for climate change adaptation and mitigation?"
[20] Ibid.

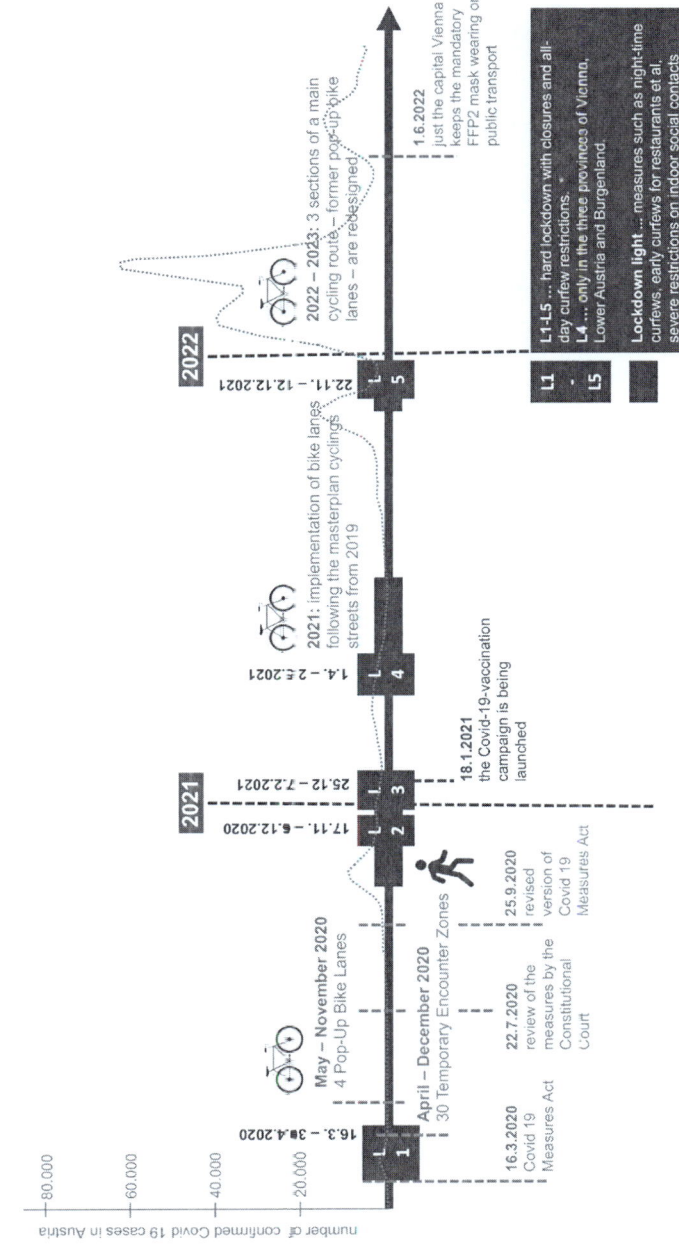

Fig. 3: The timeline from March 2020 to October 2022 shows COVID-19 case numbers (in orange), COVID-19 measures and necessary legislative changes to exit restrictions ("lockdowns"), as well as specific measures taken by Vienna for walking ("temporary encounter zones") and cycling ("pop-up cycle lanes").[21,22]

---

[21] Frey et al., „Mobilität in Wien unter COVID19. Begleituntersuchung temporäre Begegnungszonen und Pop-Up Radinfrastruktur."

[22] Vienna Center for Electoral Research, "Corona-Blog: Themenübersicht."

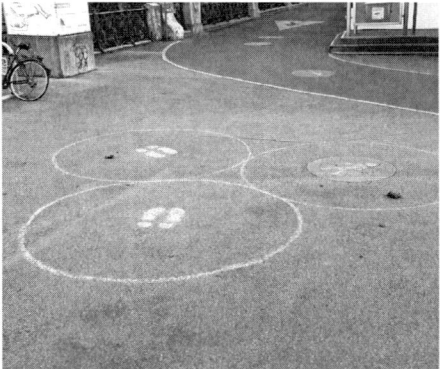
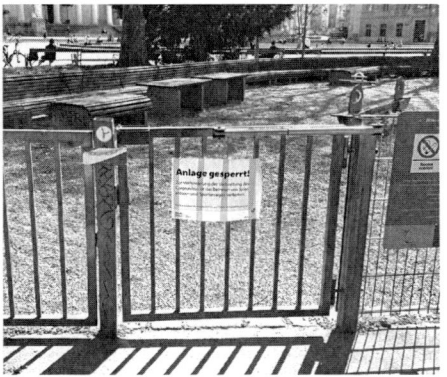

Fig. 4: Distance rule as chalk drawing, first COVID-19 lockdown, March 2020 (Photo: Irene Bittner)

Fig. 5: Closed play area in Resselpark at Karlsplatz, April 2020 (Photo: Irene Bittner)

Changes in walking, cycling and scootering in Vienna since the start of the COVID-19 pandemic

Walking in public spaces was subject to a long break in Vienna and led to a transformation of walking in the city in the medium term. While there were hardly any people on the streets at the beginning of 2020 during the first weeks of the first lockdown, walking soon experienced a real boom. Walking and strolling, as well as shopping on foot was almost the only way to move around outdoors in the city and to meet other people outside one's own household. While in 2019 the share of walking in total traffic was still only 28 percent, in 2020 it shot up to 37 percent.[23]

Transformation processes of active mobility can also be seen relatively clearly in the example of cycling in Vienna. For many years now the Vienna Urban Development Plans (STEP) have included an increase in cycling share among their various goals.[24] STEP 2015, published in 2005, set the increase from six to ten percent for the year 2015.[25] In 2015, the average share of cycling was seven percent. As such the target set in 2005 was not achieved.[26] Nevertheless,

---

[23] Mobility Agency Vienna, "Mobilität in der Corona-Krise: Wienerinnen und Wiener sind zu Fuß und per Fahrrad unterwegs."

[24] Note: The STEP functions as a strategic, city-wide planning instrument, is updated every ten years and adopted by the Vienna City Council as a legally non-binding document (policy paper) with the character of a recommendation.

[25] City of Vienna, *STEP 2015 – Stadtentwicklungsplan.*

[26] Mobility Agency Vienna, "Jahresbericht 2015."

the STEP 2025, published in 2015, set the ambitious goal of increasing cycling to twelve percent by 2025.[27] In 2019, the cycling share of seven per cent was still well below this target.[28] At the end of 2021, however, the Mobility Agency Vienna reported a "new record year" for cycling in Vienna – in the first two years of the COVID-19 pandemic, 2020 and 2021, the cycling share jumped to nine percent.[29]

In addition, even before the pandemic, e-scooters from two sharing providers became increasingly popular means of transport in Vienna. Figures relating to the use of e-scooters in Vienna are not known. It is reasonable to assume, however, that there was an increase in the years 2020 and 2021, just as with walking and cycling. An international study shows that there has been an increase in walking and cycling in many cities around the world and data from European cities such as Berlin, London and Paris indicate an increase of around 15 percent in the use of e-scooters.[30] Especially in the warm Viennese summer months of 2020, e-scooters were a popular form of micro-mobility for young people to quickly get to the next outdoor party announced at short notice. Although after the first reopenings gastronomy and trade flourished again, night gastronomy was still under restrictive curfews, first having to close by 22:00h and later 24:00h. Young people therefore met outdoors in the evening instead of in the clubs.[31] Central urban open spaces such as the Danube Canal, Karlsplatz, Heldenplatz or "Zwi-de-Mu", as a large green space between the museums along the Ringstraße is called in youth lingo, were the hotspots of a spontaneous outdoor club culture in 2020 that resisted the COVID-19 measures. E-scooters were a part of it but have also become more generally a part of the cityscape as an everyday mobility choice, even if they often mutate into obstacles for pedestrians by being carelessly parked in public spaces. In 2022, parking restrictions for e-scooters on pavements were being discussed by the City of Vienna.

---

[27] City of Vienna, "STEP 2025. Thematic Concept: Urban Mobility Plan. Together on the move."
[28] Mobility Agency Vienna, "Mobility Report 2019."
[29] Mobility Agency Vienna, "Radverkehr: 2021 neues Rekordjahr."
[30] Musselwhite, Avineri and Susilo, "Restrictions on mobility due to the coronavirus Covid19: Threats and opportunities for transport and health."
[31] Kelekhsaeva, "Transformation of Public Places in the Pandemic: The Experiences of Urbanities in St. Petersburg and Vienna."

Pop-up cycle paths and temporary encounter zones in Vienna

The pandemic led to not only restrictive measures such as lockdowns and social distancing but also opportunities for temporary, low-cost and experimental solutions to the increased need for more space for active mobility in the urban environment. What started in cities like Bogota, New York and Berlin also found its way into Vienna's cycling culture:[32,33] In 2020, four pop-up bike routes and almost 30 temporary encounter zones were introduced in Vienna. Between the end of May and the beginning of November 2020 the four pop-up bike lanes were set up in three sections – Praterstraße, Lassallestraße and Wagramer Straße – along a main cycling route to Vienna's recreational areas on the Danube and also in Hörlgasse, which has not yet received a cycle path and connects the Danube Canal with the University of Vienna.[34] The temporary encounter zones were set up between mid-April and the end of December 2020 – with an average duration of 3.75 months. The selection of the temporary encounter zones followed criteria such as narrow pavements, a high population density, no immediate proximity to parks or other green spaces, and streets with low car volumes.[35]

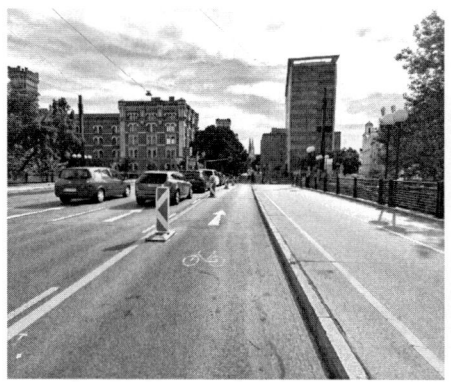

Fig. 6: Pop-up bicycle lane Hörlgasse, 2020 (Photo: Irene Bittner)

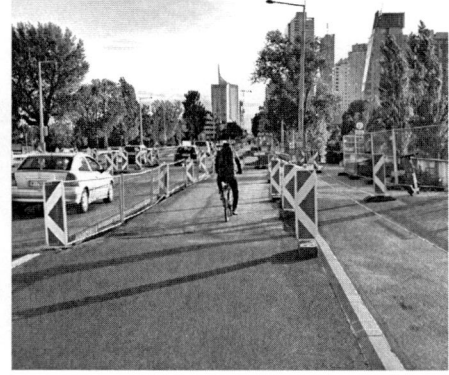

Fig. 7: Becoming a permanent bicycle lane – Pop-up bicycle lane Wagramer Straße, 2022 (Photo: Irene Bittner)

---

[32] VCÖ – Mobilität mit Zukunft, "Metropolen schaffen Platz zum Gehen und Radfahren."
[33] Kraus and Koch, "Provisional COVID-19 infrastructure induces large, rapid increases in cycling."
[34] Frey et al., „Mobilität in Wien unter COVID19. Begleituntersuchung temporäre Begegnungszonen und Pop-Up Radinfrastruktur."
[35] Ibid.

A study by the Vienna University of Technology found the temporary bike lanes and encounter zones to have had a positive impact on pedestrian and bicycle traffic. Both the pop-up bike lanes and the temporary encounter zones were better accepted when they were located alongside existing cycle routes or when a given street had previously been temporarily car-free as was the case with Hasnergasse, which had been designated a car free zone and named a "Cool Street" in summer 2019.[36] While the temporary encounter zones were in place in 2020 for the most part cars were allowed access and parking lanes for stationary traffic were maintained. Consequently, there remained a clear obstacle to the free and cross-section use of the entire street by pedestrians.[37] In the autumn of 2022, car lanes in Praterstraße, Lassallestraße and Wagramer Straße that had previously been used for the pop-up bike lanes began to be converted into permanent bike lanes.[38]

The COVID-19 crisis has made it clear that Vienna needs more space for walking, cycling and scootering

As if seen through a magnifying glass, the difficulty of finding enough space for walking, cycling and scootering in the limited street spaces of densely populated neighbourhoods has become both clearer and more explosive since the outbreak of the COVID-19 pandemic.

Even though the proportion of journeys made in traffic has returned to pre Covid-19 values time spent outdoors that became necessary in 2020 for one's own fitness and mental health and ultimately also for social contact has shown just how little space is left for walking, cycling and scootering in the streets in metropolises such as Vienna due to the huge increase in motor vehicle traffic over the decades. Studies have shown that despite the bitter background of a pandemic, it has become apparent that drastic behavioural changes towards more sustainable mobility are possible.[39,40,41] Cycling and walking have also proven to be resilient forms of mobility. After an initial general decline in overall mobility in the first weeks of the lockdown in spring 2020, active mobility

---

[36] Ibid.
[37] Ibid.
[38] Krutzler, "Radwegausbau in Wien schreitet voran, Autofahrspuren fallen weg."
[39] Kraus and Koch, "Provisional COVID-19 infrastructure induces large, rapid increases in cycling."
[40] Büchel, Marra and Corman, "COVID-19 as a window of opportunity for cycling: Evidence from the first wave."
[41] Frey et al., „Mobilität in Wien unter COVID19. Begleituntersuchung temporäre Begegnungszonen und Pop-Up Radinfrastruktur."

strongly increased in importance and measurably in numbers. In Vienna, both walking and cycling have since remained at higher volumes than in the years prior to the beginning of the pandemic.[42]

Also, in the context of the climate and energy crisis, the associated mobility turnaround and urgently needed climate change adaptation measures such as more shading by trees or cooling water elements in Vienna's streets, lessons can be learned from the experience of the COVID-19 pandemic. Already around 1900 green spaces such as Frederick L. Olmsted's Central Park in New York were considered valuable infrastructures both for the physical and mental health of the urban population (see Martin Wagner's theory on the "Sanitary Green of Cities").[43,44] From this perspective, traffic-calmed street spaces with more greenery, more places to sit and better water-storing functions could also take on the function of micro-green spaces that are well-distributed within the cityscape.

How the lessons learnt from the COVID-19 pandemic will be incorporated into mobility behaviour in the long term will presumably also depend on how consistently certain measures to reduce motor vehicle traffic and improve infrastructure for walking and cycling are pushed forward, and how much the driving wind of behavioural change caused by the pandemic can be sustained.

Bibliography

BGBl. I No. 12/2020 Federal law consolidated: Entire legal regulation for "COVID-19 Maßnahmengesetz" (Covid-19 Measures Act), version of 20.09.2022. Available at: https://www.ris.bka.gv.at/GeltendeFassung.wxe?Abfrage=Bundesnormen&Gesetzesnummer=20011073 (Accessed: 2022-09-20)

Brezina, Tadej, Ulrich Leth, and Anita Graser. "Pavement width Maps – District Comparison." Accessed November 20, 2022. www.fvv.tuwien.ac.at/institut/kompetenzfelder/fussgeher/#c13393.

Büchel, Beda, Alessio Daniele Marra, and Francesco Corman. "COVID-19 as a Window of Opportunity for Cycling: Evidence from the First Wave." *Transport policy* 116 (2022): 144–56. https://doi.org/10.1016/j.tranpol.2021.12.003.

City of Vienna. *STEP 2015 – Stadtentwicklungsplan*. 2005.

---

[42] Mobility Agency Vienna, "Mobilität in der Corona-Krise: Wienerinnen und Wiener sind zu Fuß und per Fahrrad unterwegs."
[43] Kelekhsaeva, "Transformation of Public Places in the Pandemic: The Experiences of Urbanities in St. Petersburg and Vienna."
[44] Wagner, „Das sanitäre Grün der Städte. Ein Beitrag zur Freiflächentheorie."

City of Vienna. *STEP 2025. Thematic Concept: Urban Mobility Plan. Together on the Move.* 2015.

City of Vienna, Municipal Department 18 – Urban Development and Planning. "Masterplan Fahrradstraßen." Accessed November 20, 2022. https://www.wien.gv.at/stadtentwicklung/projekte/verkehrsplanung/radwege/masterplan-fahrradstrassen.html.

Degros, Aglaée, and Eva Schwab, eds. *Territorial Justice*. GAM 15. Berlin: Jovis, 2019.

Fainstein, Susan S. *The Just City*. Ithaca, NY: Cornell University Press, 2010.

Frey, Harald, Barbara Laa, Ulrich Leth, Florian Kratochwil, and Philipp Schober. "Mobilität in Wien unter COVID19. Begleituntersuchung temporäre Begegnungszonen und Pop-up Radinfrastruktur: Durchgeführt im Auftrag der Mobilitätsagentur Wien." Accessed November 13, 2022. https://www.mobilitaetsagentur.at/wp-content/uploads/2021/02/COVID19_Mobilitaet_Wien_Endbericht_final_20201207_freyha.pdf.

Furchtlehner, Jürgen, and Lilli Lička. "Back on the Street: Vienna, Copenhagen, Munich, and Rotterdam in Focus." *Journal of Landscape Architecture* 14, no. 1 (2019): 72–83. https://doi.org/10.1080/18626033.2019.1623551.

Hartwig, Lukas, Reinhard Hössinger, Yusak Octavius Susilo, and Astrid Gühnemann. "The Impacts of a COVID-19 Related Lockdown (And Reopening Phases) On Time Use and Mobility for Activities in Austria—Results from a Multi-Wave Combined Survey." *Sustainability* 14, no. 12 (2022). https://doi.org/10.3390/su14127422.

Harvey, David. *Social Justice and the City – Revised*. Athens, US: University of Georgia Press, 2009.

Jiricka-Pürrer, Alexandra, Christiane Brandenburg, and Ulrike Pröbstl-Haider. "City Tourism Pre- and Post-Covid-19 Pandemic – Messages to Take Home for Climate Change Adaptation and Mitigation?" *Journal of Outdoor Recreation and Tourism* 31 (2020). https://doi.org/10.1016/j.jort.2020.100329.

Kelekhsaeva, Diana. "Transformation of Public Places in the Pandemic: The Experiences of Urbanities in St. Petersburg and Vienna." Working Paper. Accessed November 13, 2022. https://zdes.spbu.ru/en/53-working-papers/1498-working-papers-2048.html.

Kraus, Sebastian, and Nicolas Koch. "Provisional COVID-19 Infrastructure Induces Large, Rapid Increases in Cycling." *Proceedings of the National Academy of Sciences of the United States of America* 118, no. 15 (2021). https://doi.org/10.1073/pnas.2024399118.

Krutzler, David. "Radwegausbau in Wien schreitet voran, Autofahrspuren fallen weg." *Der Standard*, February 4, 2022. https://www.derstandard.at/story/2000133104342/radweg-ausbau-kostet-eine-autospur-auf-prater-und-lassallestrasse.

La Speranza, Marcello. *Wien im Lockdown: Zwischen Stillstand und Hoffnung*. Erfurt: Sutton, 2020.

Lehner, Daniela, Nora Heger, Jürgen Furchtlehner, and Lilli Lička, eds. *Greenspace Justice in Vienna: A Research Through Design Approach*. 2022; Proceedings of the Fábos Conference on Landscape and Greenway Planning.

Mobility Agency Vienna. "Mobilität in Der Corona-Krise: Wienerinnen und Wiener sind zu Fuß und per Fahrrad unterwegs." Accessed November 13, 2022. www.mobilitaetsagentur.at/jahresrueckblick-2020/mobilitaet-in-der-corona-krise-wienerinnen-und-wiener-sind-zu-fuss-und-per-fahrrad-unterwegs.

Mobility Agency Vienna. "Radverkehr: 2021 Neues Rekordjahr." Accessed June 10, 2022. https://www.fahrradwien.at/radfahren-in-zahlen/radzahlen-2021.

Mobility Agency Vienna. "Jahresbericht 2015." Accessed November 13, 2022. https://www.mobilitaetsagentur.at/wp-content/uploads/2016/06/MOBAG_Jahresbericht15_Web.pdf.

Mobility Agency Vienna. "Mobility Report 2019." Accessed June 11, 2022. www.mobilitaetsagentur.at/wp-content/uploads/2020/04/Mob_Report_EN_2019_RZscreen.pdf.

Musselwhite, Charles, Erel Avineri, and Yusak Susilo. "Restrictions on Mobility Due to the Coronavirus Covid19: Threats and Opportunities for Transport and Health." *Journal of transport & health* 20 (2021). https://doi.org/10.1016/j.jth.2021.101042.

Österreichische Forschungsgesellschaft Straße – Schiene – Verkehr. "Fußgängerverkehr. Richtlinien und Vorschriften für das Straßenwesen - RVS 03.02.12." Accessed November 20, 2022. www.fsv.at/shop/agliste.aspx?ID=3156234c-555a-4b8c-8a24-bb156a19e866.

Pollak, Markus, Nikolaus Kowarz, and Julia Partheymüller. "Chronologie zur Corona-Krise in Österreich – Teil 1: Vorgeschichte, der Weg in den Lockdown, die akute Phase und wirtschaftliche Folgen." Austrian Corona Panel Project (ACPP). Accessed November 20, 2022. https://viecer.univie.ac.at/corona-blog/corona-blog-beitraege/blog51/.

Reinwald, Florian, Daniela Haluza, Ulrike Pitha, and Rosemarie Stangl. "Urban Green Infrastructure and Green Open Spaces: An Issue of Social Fairness in Times of COVID-19 Crisis." *Sustainability* 13, no. 19 (2021). https://doi.org/10.3390/su131910606.

VCÖ – Mobilität mit Zukunft. "Metropolen schaffen Platz zum Gehen und Radfahren." Accessed June 10, 2022. https://www.vcoe.at/themen/mehr-platz-zum-gehen-und-radfahren.

Vienna Center for Electoral Research. "Corona-Blog: Themenübersicht." Austrian Corona Panel Project (ACPP), Accessed November 20, 2022. https://viecer.univie.ac.at/corona-.

Wagner, Martin. "Das Sanitäre Grün Der Städte. Ein Beitrag Zur Freiflächentheorie." Dissertation, Royal Technical University of Berlin, 1915.

Impact of the COVID-19 Pandemic on Public Space in Tokyo

Rinpei Miura

Introduction

Development of public space has been a concern of Tokyo urban planning since the 1970s. The COVID-19 pandemic has led to changes in the design and use of this space and developments during the pandemic may provide insight into future trends.

Since well before the advent of COVID, there have been two distinct directions with regards to public space development. One is development controlled by the state and private capital, which aims to erase boundaries between public and private space and to use public space for private purposes. The other is the creation of public space by civil society based on collaborative bottom-up processes, which is a relatively new phenomenon in Japan.

As a result of the pandemic, activities have intensified in both directions, thereby changing the character of public space. On the one hand, public spaces have been appropriated by private actors or local authorities through new use regulations and restrictions. On the other hand, citizen movements have managed to win urban spaces for public use through original and meaningful collective practices.

This study examines the impact of the COVID-19 pandemic on the development of public space in Tokyo.[1] First, we highlight the characteristics of what is called public space in Japan. We then present the contrasting trends in reshaping Tokyo's public space before and after the onset of the pandemic using

---

[1] This study is supported by a Grant-in-Aid for Scientific Research "A Sociological Study of Intersectoral Collaboration on the Reorganization of Public Space," (Research Project No. 21K13416).

two case-studies. In the first case study, we explore local government-led urban redevelopment around Shibuya Station; in the second, we examine practices steered by civil society in the Shimokitazawa area.

Public space: theoretical approaches

"Commoning", a citizen-driven practice of creating public space

Public space has been an important research topic since the late 20th century with political struggles over public space being discussed in a variety of ways in the social sciences.[2,3,4,5]

The common understanding of public space refers to an open space, such as a square, a street space, or an urban green space, which can be used by everyone. UN HABITAT's definition of public space is as follows:

"A public space refers to an area or place that is open and accessible to all peoples, regardless of gender, race, ethnicity, age, or socio-economic level. These are public gathering spaces such as plazas, squares, and parks. Connecting spaces, such as sidewalks and streets, are also public spaces."[6]

In this study, the concept of public space is approached somewhat differently. We first pose the question of whether an urban space that is not used at all can be considered a public space. In Japanese cities, many spaces are open and accessible, but few people use them. With the onset of the pandemic, many parks and squares became completely empty spaces. Open urban spaces in Japan can be considered as public spaces based on the above-mentioned criteria, but for a long time, they have not been used as such.

In recent years, however, attitudes toward urban open spaces have changed. In certain Tokyo neighbourhoods such as Shimokitazawa, residents are showing great interest in the urban space that surrounds them. Through discussions about the space, shared activities in the space, and new uses, citizens appropriate urban space and give meaning to it. In our study, we relate this phenomenon to David Harvey's concept of "urban commons". Harvey describes "commoning" as the practice of social groups taking possession of common

---

[2] Lefebvre, *Le droit à la ville*.
[3] Harvey, *Rebel Cities: From the Right to the City to the Urban Revolution*.
[4] Mitchell and Staeheli, "Clean and Safe? Property Redevelopment, Public Space, and Homelessness in Downtown San Diego."
[5] Arefi, *Deconstructing Placemaking*.
[6] https://mirror.unhabitat.org/content.asp?typeid=19&catid=508&cid=10548.

good.[7] Thus, urban commons refer to space created, managed, and used by civil society. However, since the interests of each group differ, there may be conflicts over the space. Although Harvey does not fully clarify the difference between communality and publicness, we understand publicness as a universal rule in which common interests are maximised and social legitimacy is granted.[8] Thus, public space is a space where people participate in the realisation of publicness.

Commoning is strongly related to the concept of "placemaking". The latter gained prominence in the United States in the 1960s, when theorists such as Jane Jacobs and William H. Whyte introduced new ideas about the use of city space.[9] Focusing on the social and cultural importance of vibrant neighbourhoods and inviting public spaces, they challenged modernist functionalist concepts of urban space. While commoning is the social act of negotiation, communication, and experimentation necessary to manage shared resources (commons), placemaking is the practice of commoning specifically in the context of urban space.[10]

Japanese cities and public space

Japanese architect Fumihiko Maki once argued that Japanese cities are fundamentally different from European cities, lacking above all centrality and the typical patterns of centrality such as the presence of public squares and important monuments.[11] While European cities display religious and civic power in the centre of the city[12], in Japan, important sites such as shrines and temples are located outside the cities, in areas that are difficult to see.

The historical lack of public space in Japan's cities has been discussed since the 1960s. The work of the *Toshi dezain kenkyūtai* (Urban Planning Research Group), which included architect Isozaki Arata and architectural historian Itō Teiji, emerged against the backdrop of modernist urban planning debates and

---

[7] Harvey, *Rebel Cities: From the Right to the City to the Urban Revolution*.
[8] Tanaka, *Chiiki kara umareru kokyosei; kokyosei to kyodosei no koten*.
[9] Jacobs, *The Death and Life of Great American Cities. The Failure of Town Planning*.
[10] Today, the term "placemaking" is used in many ways-not only by citizens and organizations working to improve the community, but also by planners and developers who use it as a brand to signal authenticity and quality (https://www.pps.org/article/what-is-placemaking).
[11] Maki, *City with a Hidden Past*.
[12] Jinnai, Mitsuya and Itoi, *Hiroba - Space Design Series Vol.7*.

contributed significantly to the debate on public space in Japan.[13,14] The following remarks were not aimed at reforming Japanese cities or imitating European cities, but rather at understanding the particularities of Japanese cities:

"Have there ever been public spaces in our country? This question has been asked many times by many people up to the present day, and the answer has always remained a mystery. If we are asked if there was ever an independent open space that everyone could unanimously approve of, such as the agora of ancient Greece, the piazza of medieval Italy, or the Place de la Concorde in Paris during the Baroque period, we can only answer that we have never had such a space. However, if we define a public space as something that brings people together, whether socially, economically, or politically, and if any man-made open spaces are used for that purpose, [...] then we can say that such spaces have indeed existed.

Public spaces in Japan have existed through human activities. The word "hiroba" refers not only to a physical space, but also to an artificial open space that can exist only through a social practice."[15]

According to the above arguments, the Japanese term *hiroba* cannot be equated one-to-one with Western concepts such as plaza, square, or piazza. *hiroba* are spaces that temporarily serve as hubs of religious, political and economic communication. *hiroba* are not always open spaces. In Japan, various forms of *hiroba* have existed since the Middle Ages, found temporarily at Shinto rituals at shrines deep in the mountains or at festivals in city streets.[16] *Hiroba* must therefore be understood as a dynamic process rather than a static, physical place[17], social practice being a key aspect of *hiroba*.

It is precisely this feature of social practice that necessitates the redefinition of the common concept public space. The ancient Japanese practice of citizens creating spaces for themselves through different uses, albeit temporarily, can be seen as a precursor to British geographer David Harvey's concept of "commoning". Commoning is not only about social practice in space, it also involves the political process of debate and confrontation about the nature of space. Against the backdrop of a predominantly capitalist use of urban space, the countervailing practice of commoning, aimed at realising publicness by civil society, is becoming increasingly important.[18]

---

[13] Urban Design Body, "Nihon no Hiroba."
[14] Miura, *Hiroba no kukan kosei*.
[15] Urban Design Body, "Nihon no Hiroba," 76.
[16] Urban Design Body, "Nihon no Hiroba," 77–88.
[17] Okabe, "Dynamic Spaces with Subjective Depth. The Public Space in Monsoon Asia," 158.
[18] Harvey, *Rebel Cities: From the Right to the City to the Urban Revolution*.

Japanese modernist after-war urban planning (from the mid-1950s to the mid-1970s) in particular has made it difficult for citizens to create their own public space. The conversion of streets into monofunctional traffic areas at that time, the zoning principle[19] applied at that time, but also increasingly complex ownership structures made flexible use of urban space almost impossible. From today's perspective, Japan's Public Property Management Act also complicates the creation of spaces where users can set their own rules and manage and operate the space themselves. A law reform drafted in 2003[20] promotes the opening of public property and services to the private sector, with the aim of boosting the Japanese economy.[21]

In response to this development, both the public and private sector began to pay more attention to the relation between urban space and civil society. At the same time, urban redevelopment initiatives driven by the state and private capital have been launched, with the aim to use urban spaces that could be public spaces, for private purposes.

The creation of public space: policies and movements

The state-led "Urban Renaissance Policies"

Since the late 2010s, foreign and especially American "placemaking" projects have been used as models for new projects in Tokyo.[22] Today, the Japanese state encourages rather than inhibits civil society involvement in planning. Until recently, however, awareness of the social dimension of space was much lower in Japan than in the United States.

One of the reasons for this reorientation in urban planning was the desire to reposition Tokyo in international city competition. At the beginning of the 1990s, Tokyo was ranked as a global city alongside London and New York[23], but the economic crisis after the bubble economy burst at the end of the 1990s had weakened this position.[24] As a partial measure, since the early 2000s, the Koizumi government has focused its efforts on the regeneration

---

[19] Zoning is a land use principle originated from the fourth CIAM of architecture, published in the "Athens charter" of 1933, that provides for the demixing of urban functions in a delimited urban area.
[20] https://www8.cao.go.jp/kisei/en/index.html#taken.
[21] Sonoda, *Pureisumeikingu akuteibitei · fuasuto no toshi dezain*.
[22] Ibid.
[23] Sassen, *The Global City: New York, London, Tokyo*.
[24] Machimura, *Back to Voices of the City*.

of Tokyo's urban centres. One of the goals of the so-called *Urban Renaissance Policy* program introduced at that time, was to improve public space to attract private and human capital. In a report on public-private partnerships in urban planning, the Ministry of Land, Infrastructure, Transport and Tourism (MLIT) clarified its intention to "actively allow the private sector to engage in profitable activities in public spaces, creating a revitalisation and an improved management of urban spaces"[25]. In 2014, the MLIT organised a symposium on the subject of "placemaking" to find new ideas for designing public space.[26] With the project *Public Spaces that create and improve Liveliness and Vitality*, the MLIT aimed to support projects in the initial phase with public funds so that they can later develop into subsidy-free projects. In 2020, the Road Traffic Act[27] was amended with regard to the revitalisation of road spaces. In specific areas of designated streets, standards for shopping and advertising scaffolding occupancy were relaxed. The system also allows for flexible change, moving away from car-oriented use in the past to creative use by people[28].

The *Urban Renaissance Policy* is merely a top-down neoliberal approach, with the government granting exceptions in the form of *Tokku* districts. These are specific areas where measures such as the relaxation of regulations are applied by the government in order to encourage economic activities and businesses.

Despite the stated goal of "creating viability"[29], the focus is primarily on economic aspects and the purpose of strengthening Tokyo's position in global competition. While policymakers argue that this type of placemaking represents a new way of urban development[30], in reality it is capital-oriented spatial planning under the guise of placemaking.

---

[25] MLIT, "Survey on the Promotion of Town Development Utilizing the Public-Private Partnership System."
[26] MLIT.
[27] https://elaws.e-gov.go.jp/document?lawid=335AC0000000105.
[28] The Demonstration project shows traits of American 'New Urbanism' principles. However, since Japanese cities are not overly dependent on the automobiles, models such as 'New Urbanism', which place all amenities within walking distance and push the automobile into the background, are rarely considered in practice or research. (Nakajima, "Nyuabanizumu naki nihon no takuteikaru abanizumu.")
[29] Ibid.
[30] Ibid.

The creation of "pseudo-public" and "pseudo-private" spaces

However, not only public but also private space is undergoing alteration in connection with the above-mentioned urban development policies. According to the common understanding of space, private space is separate from public space. Nevertheless, one can observe that the boundaries between public and private space in Tokyo are becoming increasingly blurred. This development can be seen against the background of Mitchell's and Staehli's discussion on "pseudo-public" and "pseudo-private" spaces (2006). "Pseudo-public" spaces refers to spaces that were originally public (e.g., parks) but which have since been redeveloped for private purposes and are now more likely to be private spaces. "Pseudo-private" spaces refers to spaces that are private (e.g., shopping malls) but which justify their existence by satisfying social needs and laying claim to be public spaces.

Since the 2000s, the above-mentioned state-led neoliberal *Urban Renaissance Policy* has led to gentrification-like phenomena in Tokyo's urban centres.[31] This state-led development policy aims to create large-scale commercial facilities, office buildings, hotels or tower condominiums near important urban hubs such as stations, but in doing so, pseudo-public space and pseudo-private space, in which public space is used to gain profit, are proliferating. The large-scale redevelopment of Tokyo's urban centres which took place in preparation for the 2020 Olympics is an example of this policy.

Such state-led transformations of urban space were not halted by the onset of the pandemic. On the contrary, they accelerated, due in part to the government's call for self-restraint and the resulting cancellation of all civic activities in public space.

Response of Japanese society to the pandemic

The government's call for self-restraint

The pandemic hit Japan in March 2020 and on April 7 the Japanese government declared its first state of emergency under the Law Concerning Special Measures against the New Coronavirus, passed on March 13, 2020. The emergency declaration was not a draconian measure that banned movement or business, as was

---

[31] Miura, "Rethinking Gentrification and the Right to the City: The Process and Effect of the Urban Social Movement Against Redevelopment in Tokyo.'

the case in other countries[32]. Since there is no legal basis for a lockdown in Japan, local authorities can only urge the population not to leave their communities. The contradiction in the meaning of the term "request for self-restraint" is a clear indication of the predicament of Japan's infection control measures. While the content of the "request for self-restraint" was to be considered by each local government head, the responses of all local governments were based on the government's principle of avoiding gatherings of people. Emergency restrictions were imposed on the communities with the largest number of cases. Tokyo, the most populous area, was the target of emergency restrictions every time.

Mutual surveillance among citizens

Control over urban spaces was made possible not only by governmental exhortations but also by mutual surveillance. Fear of unknown infectious diseases led people to crack down privately, attacking people, stores, and vendors who did not comply with the local government's call for self-restraint. This led to the blaming of children playing in parks and other public spaces, among other examples.[33] Such accusers were derided on the Internet as "self-restraint police".[34] Nevertheless, mutual surveillance conducted anonymously also had some influence on discourses about public space.

A society of mutual surveillance – what Jock Young calls an "exclusionary society" – existed before the pandemic.[35] However, it appears that the pandemic has exacerbated this phenomenon, facilitating new regulations in public spaces that exclude certain social groups.

Miyashita Park: from public to pseudo-public space

The Miyashita Park project described below is the result of a state-led initiative that promoted the transformation of an originally public space into a pseudo-public space. The completion of the project, but also the reorganisation of the management and use of the new urban space, took place a few months after the beginning of the pandemic.

---

[32] Based on information from the Cabinet Secretariat's official website on countermeasures against infectious diseases.
(https://corona.go.jp/emergency/.)
[33] Yomiuri Newspaper.
[34] Matsubara, "'Jishuku-keisatsu (self-restraint police)' under the COVID-19 pandemic in Japan Focusing on transformation of discursive space."
[35] Young, *The Exclusive Society: Social Exclusion, Crime and Difference in Late Modernity.*

Shibuya Ward development policies

Shibuya Ward is located in the southwestern part of Tokyo, adjacent to the central business district and one of the three major subcentres. It is a downtown area and an office district with many high-end residential areas in its vicinity. The scramble crossing in front of Shibuya Station is a famous tourist spot both in Japan and abroad and, as a district frequented by many young people, it is an area that has continued to change with the trends of each era.

The area shown in Figure 1 is an area around Shibuya Station which is undergoing redevelopment (scheduled to be completed by 2024), most of which has been designated as a *Tokku* district under the urban renewal policy, allowing the construction of high-rise buildings.

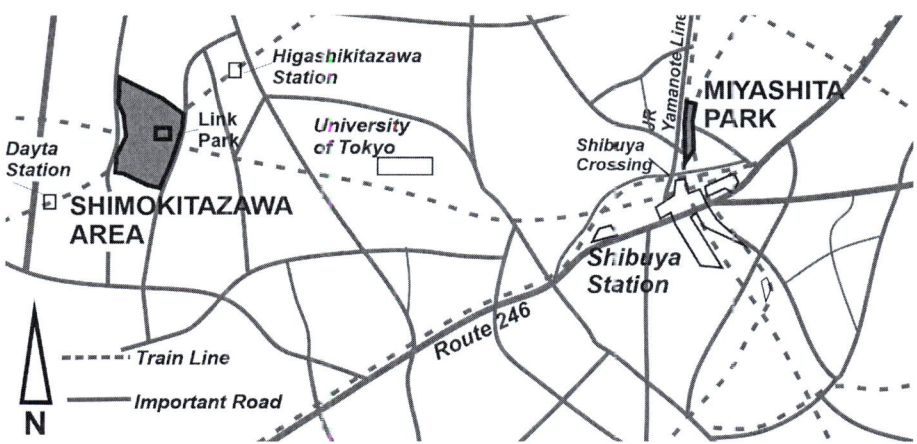

Fig. 1: Location of Miyashita Park und Shimokitazawa Area
(Illustration: Rinpei Miura)

Since 2003, the Shibuya Ward government has repeatedly submitted development plans. Central to these plans is Shibuya Station – considered to be the face of the Shibuya district. The city's rationale for the plans was not only to improve urban space for local residents but also to position Shibuya in international urban competition.

In the *Basic Concept* of 2016, Shibuya Ward is described as a "mature international city" that can be ranked with London, Paris, and New York.[36] "Maturi-

---

[36] Shibuya Ward, *Shibuya City – the Basic Concept*.

ty" in this context is interpreted as a high level of international competitiveness that is linked to a "strong regional character", enabling residents of the district to live there with pride. Strong regional character is understood to be the concentration of commercial and entertainment facilities, content industries, and cultural and exchange functions, as well as the diversity of visitors from Japan and abroad. In 2020, the Shibuya Ward government issued a development concept entitled *2020 Creative City Shibuya* aiming to "transmit Shibuya's culture to the world" through redevelopment projects.[37] The same year, the Shibuya Ward elaborated the *Shibuya Ward Urban Development Master Plan,* emphasising the need for more public space for activities that lead to community building.[38] According to the plan, any open and "open-space-like" space is considered to be public space.

In 2021, the government introduced the *Shibuya Smart City Basic Policy*, which is characterised by the idea of "diversity". The policy is about creating urban spaces, whether public or private, where a variety of people spend time, and interaction and connections occur. Even though this seems to be a noble goal, the question arises whether the kind of diversity found in public space can be reproduced in private space.

One of the projects carried out on the basis of the above-mentioned strategies is Miyashita Park, which has attracted much attention both in Japan and abroad. Not only the design of the stores in the commercial facility, but also the fact that a public park was transformed into a large-scale commercial facility, raised a debate about the meaning and nature of public space.

The transformation of Miyashita Park into a commercial facility

As of 2017, the new Miyashita Park Development Project sealed off the park, so that a complex with a hotel and commercial facilities could be built there; the park's functions (green space, seats accessible for everyone) were to be moved to the roof of the building along with sports facilities. Completed in July 2020, Miyashita Park is now a three-story, large-scale commercial building with a rooftop hotel, a café, and a rooftop park. The first-floor houses luxury brand stores such as Louis Vuitton, Gucci, Balenciaga, Prada, and Coach, the second and third floors are occupied by a wide variety of restaurants, apparel stores, and retail stores. As the photos clearly show, it is not possible to even guess that this place, now managed and operated by Mitsui Real Estate, used to be a public park.

---

[37] Shibuya Ward, *2020 Creative City Shibuya.*
[38] Shibuya Ward, *Shibuya City Urban Development Master Plan.*

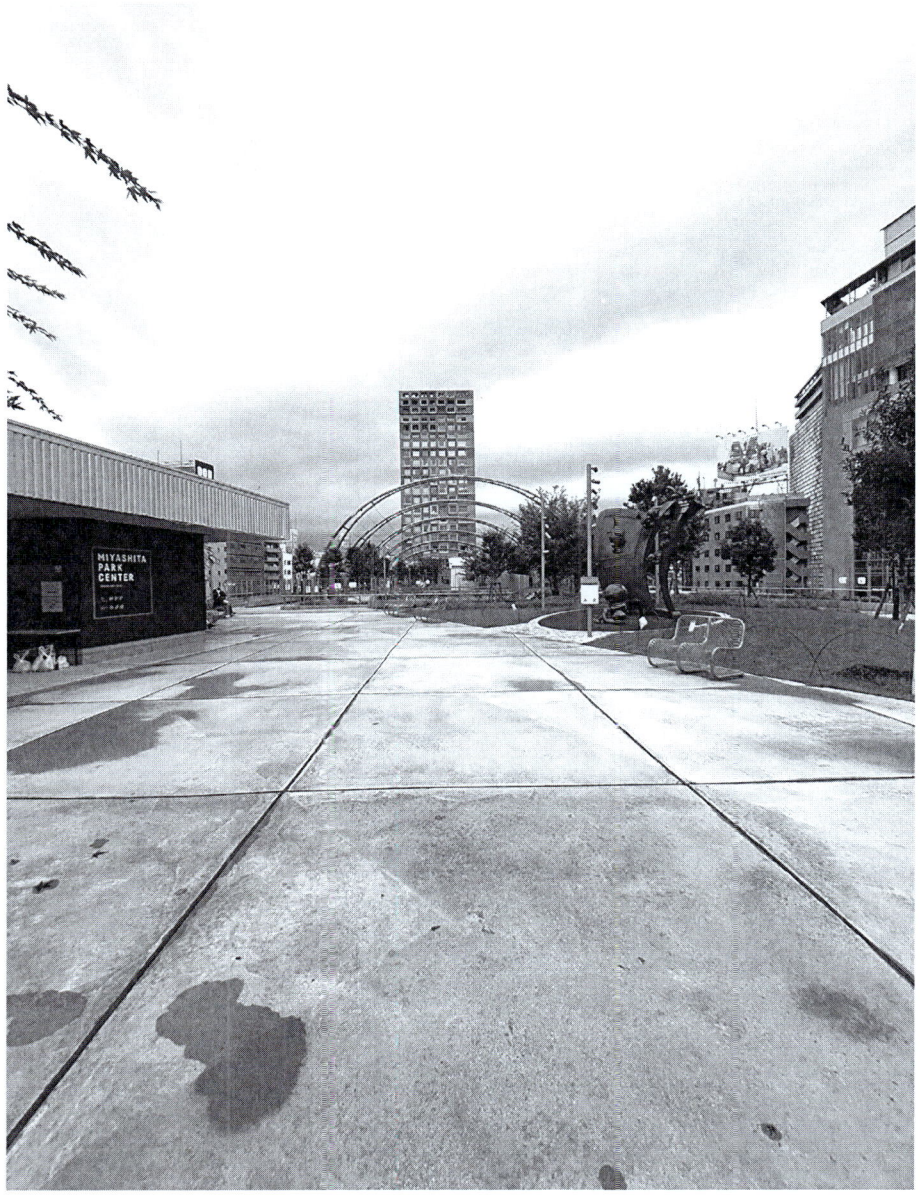

Fig. 2: Rooftop Park of new Miyashita Park (Photo: Rinpe Miura)

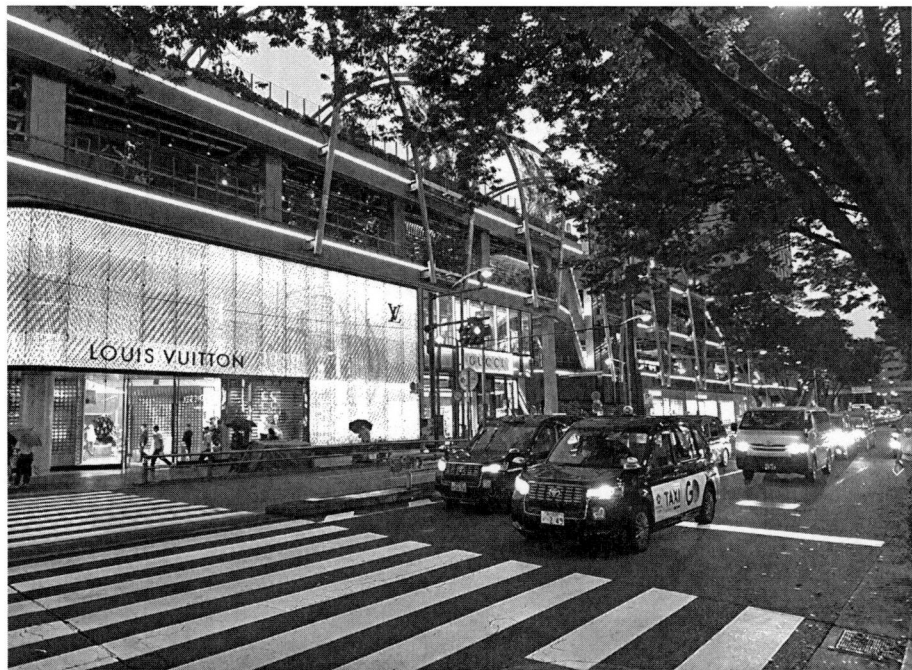

Fig. 3: Exterior view of new Miyashita Park (Photo: Rinpei Miura)

On the website of Mitsui Real Estate it says: "Miyashita Park is a new social hub that embraces a diverse community"[39]. The notion of "diversity" that is also addressed by Shibuya Ward's *Smart City Policy* refers to customers of the commercial establishments and, in this respect, does not bring any novelty.[40] True diversity, which is characterised among other things by a variety of people from different social backgrounds, is scarce and additionally challenged by the pandemic.

The pandemic and the accelerated exclusion of homeless people

As in other commercial establishments, infection control measures have been thoroughly enforced at Miyashita Park since the pandemic began. Many stores require customers to sanitise their hands upon entering, customers are asked not to sit next to each other on benches placed inside the facilities or in the parks. Space is thoroughly managed so that situations with high human density are avoided as

---

[39] https://www.mitsuifudosan.co.jp/english/corporate/news/2020/0120/.
[40] Wakabayashi, *Moru ka suru toshi to shakai*.

much as possible. Control through official rules extend to the parts of the parks where a variety of uses were possible before the reconstruction and the pandemic. Mutual surveillance provides additional control at a low-threshold level.

The following prohibitions are posted at the park entrances:

- Damaging or defacing the facilities
- Use of fire
- Displaying advertisements
- Loud music, chorus, or speeches
- Distribution of leaflets, goods, food, or drinks
- Installation of structures
- Lying down
- Prolonged use of benches

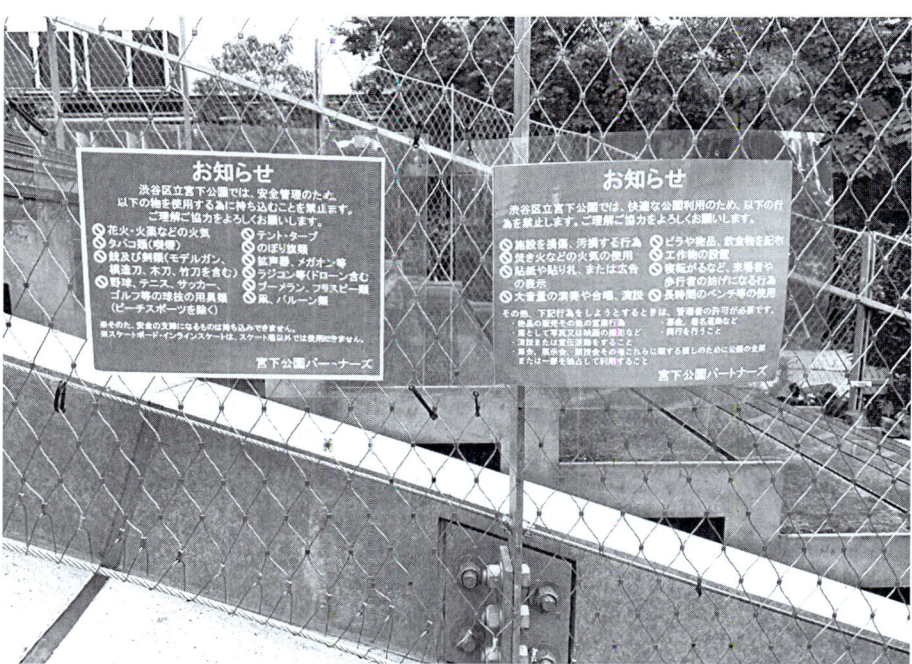

Fig. 4: Prohibited activities in Miyashita Park (Photo: Rinpei Miura)

The prohibitions were imposed together with the COVID measures by the Miyashita Park administration[41] in the summer of 2020. The administration of the park operates almost exclusively along private-sector lines. Yet, Miyashita Park houses not only private facilities, but also a park that in its original form was a space for homeless people. Although the management does not specifically state that homeless people are prohibited from entering the rooftop-park, it excludes them by banning activities they engaged in at this location before the building was completed.

The new opening hours of the park were partly justified by the risk of infection. The rooftop-park is accessible from 8:00 am. to 11:00 pm and closed during the year-end and New Year's Day, while commercial facilities are open on these holidays. The former park used to be a place to sleep for the homeless, the hours of the new rooftop park do not meet their needs. A ban on using the park during the night and on holidays can be life-threatening.

Since the beginning of the pandemic, there has been little support for homeless people in Miyashita Park nor has help been available due to concerns about the risk of infection. However, in the summer of 2022, concerned groups asked the Shibuya Municipal Government to provide a new space where those in need could find refuge during the extremely hot days and nights.[42]

The pandemic is challenging publicness

The case of Miyashita Park may be an indication of how Tokyo's public space will be treated in the future. The proliferation of pseudo-public spaces through redevelopment in central Tokyo attracts a diverse range of visitors, creates various activities, and gives birth to a bustling atmosphere, but these are places that can be used only by those who have been selected by the market. Socially vulnerable groups are excluded in various ways.

There have been various media reports on the increasing number of people losing their jobs and of people falling into poverty due to the COVID-19 epidemic. According to a support group in Tokyo, the number of people using food banks increased from 100 to about 500 between the start of the pandemic and summer 2022.[43] In this light, a new political conflict over the nature of public space may emerge in the future. In fact, advocacy groups have been

---

[41] The operator Miyashita Park Partners consists of Mitsui Real Estate managing and operating the commercial part of   Miyashita Park and Seibu Landscaping, which is responsible for the park management and operation.
[42] Tokyo Newspaper.
[43] Asahi Newspaper.

persistently campaigning against the Miyashita project, and this is likely to gain momentum as poverty increases.

The pandemic has certainly led to a more accelerated exclusion of the poor from public space, while simultaneously making political conflicts more apparent. Debates may arise about the definition of public space and whether today's Miyashita Park is more desirable for urban life than a space like the former Miyashita Park. Further, there is the question of who designs, manages, and operates public space. The pseudo-public space represented by Miyashita Park is managed by local government and private companies, with little room for civil society to intervene. Commoning activities are very weak.

Commoning before and during the pandemic in the Shimokitazawa Area

Shimokitazawa Area's development policy

Near the new pseudo-public space in Shibuya Ward, a civil society-led initiative to create a better public space has recently been launched in Shimokitazawa, Setagaya Ward. With about 920,000 residents, Setaga is the most populous administrative district in Tokyo. Shimokitazawa is located in the northeastern part of Setagaya, 10 minutes by train from Shibuya Station (Fig. 1). The local government considers Shimokitazawa to be one of the three major commercial/business centres of the Ward, along with Futako-Tamagawa and Sangen-Jaya.[44]

Like Shibuya, Shimokitazawa also experienced development, but in this case it was not the local government but the Tokyo Metropolitan Government and the MLIT which took the lead. In the early 2000s, the so-called *Grade Separation Project* was initiated. The removal of existing railroad tracks (by raising them or moving them underground) was intended to free up space not only for commercial and residential buildings, but also for new roads and, especially, new public spaces. In 2003, the public authorities announced that the Odakyu line would be moved underground, and the level crossings would be eliminated. These were the basic conditions for the realisation of the project.[45]

---

[44] Setagaya, *Setagaya Ward Urban Development Policy*.
[45] Miura, *Kyosei no toshi shakaigaku – shimokitazawa saikaihatsu no naka de kangaeru*.

Commoning by Shimokita Ring[46]

In 2016, the administration of Setagaya Ward established the *Shimokita Ring Citizens' Forum*[47] to discuss possible uses of the former railroad site which extended about 2 km from Daita Station to Higashikitazawa Station. The goal of the forum was to gather a wide range of ideas concerning the future public space and with this in mind various subcommittees on specific topics were formed.

The land use policy for the vacated railroad land was determined by the Setagaya Ward administrative body and Odakyu Electric Railway Co, Ltd, who own the rights to the land. Their land use plan called, amongst other things, for the completion of the large station forecourt. The "Green Subcommittee" and the "Station Square Subcommittee" pointed out problems with the land use plan such as the lack of both green and open spaces and the lack of transparency concerning the management of these spaces. As an alternative project, the Green Subcommittee proposed to expand green spaces. This suggestion was the result of a survey of residents. After minor modifications and several rounds of discussion, the subcommittee's proposals were accepted, and the original plan was revised.

The Station Square Subcommittee addressed the development and design of the square in front of Shimokitazawa Station, which until 2020 was unused wasteland waiting for a makeover. The goal was to make the square a space where pedestrians had priority over cars in the long term. The first step was to convert the wasteland into an area that could be used by all road users on a trial basis until construction would begin. A part of the unused construction site area north of the station was to become an experimental public space. In the so-called *Link Park*, a space to connect people with each other, different temporary uses were to be made possible (Fig. 5). The experience gained from *Link Park* should then be incorporated into the permanent concept of the whole station square.

---

[46] The analysis of the Shimokitazawa area activities is based on observation and interviews by the author.
[47] Previous name: 'Kitazawa PR Strategy Conference'.

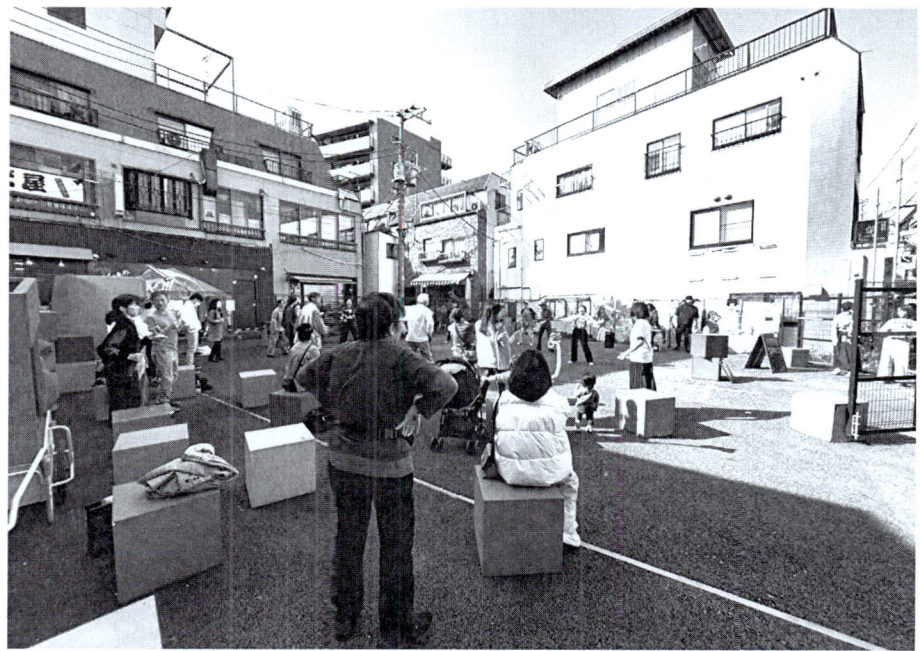

Fig. 5: Link Park, temporary uses (Photo: Rinpei Miura)

Commoning Confronts Pandemic

After the government declared a state of emergency in April 2020, the activities of the Green Subcommittee and other Shimokita Ring subcommittees, as well as activities in *Link Park*, were cancelled or postponed. Some community activities and meetings continued online.[48] An important aspect of commoning, however, is physical meetings and social interaction in public space. The Shimokita Ring slowly began to resume its activities in public space only in the summer of 2021, when the last emergency declaration was lifted.

One particularly active group was the Green Subcommittee which had been reorganised as an incorporated association in January 2020, under a new organisation called the "Shimokita Gardening Subcommitee". In the spring of 2022, when a planned raised bed and other green spaces were completed, members began to actively participate in the maintenance and management

---

[48] Koyama, "Korona ka ni okeru machizukuri katsudo no keizoku to tenkai ni kansuru ichi kosatsu."

of the green spaces. The Gardening Subcommittee organised events such as an open house with workshops on the green space, where people could drink locally produced herbal tea and buy *Shimokita Honey*. Furthermore, it started an initiative that consisted of accepting plants that had grown too large from private homes, with the aim of repotting and selling them. In addition, it established the *Shimokita Garden School*, which teaches local citizens how to protect and maintain the green spaces throughout the former railroad area, as well as green spaces in the city in general. The Gardening Subcommittee views the community's greenery as a shared resource (commons) and encourages the entire community to participate in the cyclical process of planting, tending, harvesting and returning plants to the soil.

The activities of the Station Square Subcommittee were largely suspended during the pandemic, which had serious consequences for the development of the square. During the first month of the pandemic, the Setagaya Ward administration developed the Station Square into a road area dedicated solely to motorised traffic, as originally planned. This was not in line with the subcommittee's concept of public space that could be freely used by pedestrians. No compromises were sought for this traffic node, in fact the gap between the ideal of public space and the built reality at the station square grew. The pandemic and the loss of control of the subcommittee had brought the activities of this weaker of the two communities of interest to a standstill, playing into the hands of the top-down planners.

Nevertheless, the subcommittee is actively looking at alternatives. One suggestion is to lay artificial turf on the Shimokitazawa station square, following the example of another site in Tokyo. This approach is intended to stimulate participatory processes and strengthen citizen autonomy – citizens should realise that urban space is their own space and experiment with new uses.

Meanwhile, commoning practices have achieved some success in the *Link Park project*. The Station Square Subcommittee was able to open *Link Park* as early as summer 2021. Since then, various events have taken place, such as concerts, festivals, flea-markets and other activities related to a subsistence-economy, which has become more important since the pandemic. A Facebook page has been set up where events are announced, and citizens are invited to participate and to communicate their ideas. In the summer of 2022, the subcommittee started to hold events in Link Park, where citizens can discuss their ideas for using public space.

Since there are few areas in Shimokitazawa where people can sit and children can play, the subcommittee has set up wooden boxes and laid artificial turf for children to play on.

Conclusion

Even before the COVID-19 pandemic, Tokyo was experiencing a steady shrinking of public space through the creation of pseudo-private and pseudo-public spaces. However, the pandemic has accelerated this development. Citizens' efforts to create and maintain public space form a countermovement to top-down processes and developments driven by private capital. The appropriation of open urban space by citizens through meaningful collective activities, which can also be referred to as "commoning", attracted public attention in that citizens' participation in planning processes was unusual in Japan until recently. The Shimokita Ring, a citizen's forum in Shimokitazawa, created with the aim of shaping public space by commoning activities, is emblematic of the new enthusiasm of Tokyo residents to participate in the development of their own urban environment.

The state of emergency and the fear of the risk of infection related to COVID-19 have led to the cancellation of many crucial commoning activities. This circumstance has facilitated the takeover of disputed public space by private investors, as illustrated by the example of the new Miyashita Park, where new usage rules are being established and controlled by private operators. Furthermore, local governments have profited from the pandemic by determining the use of urban space without seeking dialogue with citizens. Shimokitazawa Station Square for example, was transformed into a monofunctional traffic area against the will of local citizens after the cessation of Shimokita Ring activities due to the pandemic.

However, there are areas where commoning activities have yielded concrete results. In Shomikitazawa, various ideas of the Shimokita Gardening Subcommittee have been realised, and Link-Park was able to open a year after the outbreak of the pandemic. Since then, these spaces have become very popular, characterised by diverse usage and original actions.

Recently, and especially since the beginning of the pandemic, the subsistence economy has gained attention in Japan. There seems to be an increasing consensus that what constitutes human dignity and human relations cannot be based solely on the logic of the market. Exchange relationships in the non-market economy are part of commoning activities. The expansion of public spaces, where people also engage in activities and exchanges that do not depend on the market, will be increasingly important for mutual support and local communities in the future.

Commoning is proving to be a key factor in countering shrinkage of public space and irreversible developments. Participatory civil society-driven practices of space creation are crucial aspects of urban development and should be adopted by all local communities, alongside market and subsistence economies initiatives. However, like all civil society activities, commoning needs to be constantly reviewed. The experience of the pandemic and the desire to control infection in particular may lead to the emergence of control practices similar to those in pseudo-public and pseudo-private spaces. The creation and management of public spaces always carries the risk of excluding certain social groups, groups that are "different". This risk was amplified by the pandemic.

Bibliography

https://elaws.e-gov.go.jp/document?lawid=335AC0000000105.

https://www8.cao.go.jp/kisei/en/index.html#taken.

https://www.mitsuifudosan.co.jp/english/corporate/news/2020/0120/. Accessed November 17, 2022.

https://corona.go.jp/emergency. Accessed October 10, 2022.

https://mirror.unhabitat.org/content.asp?typeid=19&catid=508&cid=10548.

The Politics of Public Space. New York: Routledge, 2006, 2006.

Yomiuri Newspaper, Dema kakusan kyaku ga gekigen, May 13, 2020.

Asahi Newspaper, Tomaranu bukkadaka shien girigiri, June 7, 2022.

Tokyo Newspaper, Nojukusha ni your no hinan basho o, July 13, 2022.

Arefi, Mahyar. *Deconstructing Placemaking*. New York: Routledge, 2014.

Cassegard, Carl. "Public Space in Recent Japanese Political Thought and Activism: From the Rivers and Lakes to Miyashita Park." *Japan Studies* 31, no. 3 (2011): 405–22.

Dimmer, Christian. "Miyashita Park, Tokyo – Contested Visions of Public Space in Contemporary Urban Japan." In *City Unsilenced: Urban Resistance and Public Space in the Age of Shrinking Democracy*. Edited by Jeffrey Hou and Sabine Knierbein, 199–213. New York, NY: Routledge, 2017.

Harvey, David. *Rebel Cities: From the Right to the City to the Urban Revolution*. London: Verso, 2012.

Illich, Ivan. *Shadow Work*. Open Forum Series. Boston, London: Marion Boyars, 1981.

Jacobs, Jane. *The Death and Life of Great American Cities. The Failure of Town Planning*. New York: Vintage Books, 1961.

Jinnai, Hidenobu; Mitsuya, Toru and Itoi, Takao. *Hiroba - Space design series. Vol.7.* Nagoya: Shin nihon houki publishing, 1994.

Kimura, Masato. "Privatization and Protest of Commons: On the Gentrification and Homeless Movement in Shibuya." *Space, Society and Geographical Thought* 22 (2019): 139–56.

Koyama, Hiromi. "Korona ka ni okeru machizukuri katsudo no keizoku to tenkai ni kansuru ichi kosatsu." *Japan Association of Regional and Community Studies Annual Report.* 34 (2022): 41–56.

Lefebvre, Henri. *Le droit à la ville.* Paris : Anthropos, 1963.

Machimura, Takashi. *Back to Voices of the City.* Tokyo: Yuhikaku Publisihing, 2020.

Maki, Fumihiko, ed. *City with a Hidden Past.* Tokyo: Kashima Publishing, 1980.

Matsubara, Yu. "'Jishuku-keisatsu (self-restraint police)' under the COVID-19 pandemic in Japan Focusing on transformation of discursive space." *Disaster and Kyosei* 5, no. 1 (2021): 13–27.

Mitchell, Don, and Lynn A. Staeheli. "Clean and Safe? Property Redevelopment, Public Space, and Homelessness in Downtown San Diego." In *The Politics of Public Space.* New York: Routledge, 2006.

Miura, Rinpei. *Kyosei no toshi Shakaigaku - Shimokitazawa Saikaihatsu no naka de kangaeru.* Tokyo: Shinyosha publishing, 2016.

Miura, Rinpei. "Rethinking Gentrification and the Right to the City: The Process and Effect of the Urban Social Movement Against Redevelopment in Tokyo." *International Journal of Japanese Sociology* 30, no. 1 (2021): 64–79.

Miura, Rinpei, and Toru Takeoka, eds. *Henyo suru toshi no yukue.* Bunyusha publishing, 2020.

MLIT. "Survey on the Promotion of Town Development Utilizing the Public-Private Partnership System." Accessed October 10, 2022. https://www.mlit.go.jp/common/000989644.pdf.

Najakima, Naoto. "Nyuabanizumu naki nihon no takuteikaru abanizumu." In *Rui Et Al. Eds, Tactical Urbanism. Gakugei Publishing,* 46–53., 2021.

Okabe, Akiko. "Dynamic Spaces with Subjective Depth. The Public Space in Monsoon Asia." *kult-ur revista interdisciplinària sobre la cultura de la ciutat* 4, no. 7 (2017): 151–64. https://doi.org/10.6035/Kult-ur.2017.4.7.6.

Sassen, Saskia. *The Global City: New York, London, Tokyo* Princeton, N.J.: Princeton University Press, 1991.

Setagaya Ward. *Setagaya Ward Urban Development Policy.* 2014. https://www.city.setagaya.lg.jp/mokuji/sumai/001/001/d00124102.html.

Shibuya Ward. *Guide Plan 21 for Development of Shibuya Station Area.* 2003. https://www.city.shibuya.tokyo.jp/assets/detail/files/kurashi_machi_pdf_machi_21_gaiyo.pdf.

Shibuya Ward. *Shibuya City - the Basic Concept.* 2016. https://www.city.shibuya.tokyo.jp/assets/kusei/000054391.pdf.

Shibuya Ward. *2020 Creative City Shibuya.*, 2020. https://www.seisakukikaku.metro.tokyo.lg.jp/basic-plan/future-vision/pdf/3siryo3.pdf.

Shibuya Ward. *Shibuya City Urban Development Master Plan*. 2020. https://www.city.shibuya.tokyo.jp/assets/com/000048423.pdf.

Shibuya Ward. *Shibuya Smart City Basic Policy.* 2021. https://shibuya-data.jp/pdf/shibuya_smartcity_basicpolicy_all.pdf.

Sonobe, Mashisa. *Sai majutsuka suru toshi no shakaigaku.* Kyoto: Mineruba shobo head office, 2014.

Sonoda, Satoshi. *Pureisumeikingu akuteibitei · fuasuto no toshi dezain.* Tokyo: Gakugei publishing, 2019.

Tanaka, Shigeyoshi. *Chiiki kara umareru kokyosei; kokyosei to kyodosei no koten.* Kyoto: Mineruba shobo head office, 2010.

Urban Design Body. "Nihon no Hiroba." *Kenchiku bunka* 298 (1971): 73–171.

Wakabayashi, Mikio, ed. *Moru Ka Suru Toshi to Shakai.* Tokyo: NTT Publishing, 2013.

Wirth, Louis. *Urbanism as a Way of Life.* (American Journal of Sociology) Vol 44 July 1938. [Chicago], 1938.

Young, Jock. *The Exclusive Society: Social Exclusion, Crime and Difference in Late Modernity.* London, Thousand Oaks, Calif: SAGE, 1999.

Yuasa, Makoto. *Han hinkon - suberi dai shakai kara no dasshutsu.* Tokyo: Iwanami Publishing, 2008.

CHAPTER 3:

Public Transport Amid and After the Crisis

Public Transport in Vienna and Tokyo Amid and After the COVID-19 Pandemic

Takeru Shibayama

Introduction

During the early stage of the COVID-19 pandemic when the characteristics of the virulence of SARS-CoV2 were less well-known and no vaccination was available, many governments adopted a containment strategy with the restriction of human mobility placed at the centre of it. The idea reflected the respiratory nature of the disease: by limiting human contact, the spread of the virus would be slowed, leading to fewer cases and thus to less pressure on the health care system and fewer fatalities.

Under this strategy, many governments required or recommended people to stay at home with only a few exceptions so that people's mobility was restricted to an absolute minimum. Workplaces, schools, stores, restaurants, leisure facilities and other everyday destinations were closed, and the use of online alternatives were strongly encouraged wherever possible. Where human contact was unavoidable, maintaining a physical distance of 1.5 to 2 m was enforced in order to reduce the chance of viral transmissions – often referred to as "social distancing". Additional preventative measures were also introduced, in particular the use of face coverings, with some countries making FFP2 masks compulsory.

In addition to such restrictions, placing those infected with the disease in quarantine, as well as testing those people who may have been infected was also placed at the centre of the containment strategy. So-called contact tracing – the identification of all those who had come into contact with an infected person during the viral incubation and symptomatic stages – was the first step.

This also allowed governments to track the number of cases, which in turn served as the basis for decision-making on containment policies.

Restrictions on movement and further containment measures directly affected the transport sector. Travel demands plummeted overnight during the restrictions on mobility, and the transport sector was also required to respond to the aforementioned containment measures.

Means of transport are generally categorised into private and public, as well as those having an intermediate character. Private transport is characterised by the operation of one's own vehicle such as a bicycle or a car, or travel on foot. Intermediate means include taxis and car-sharing: the use is private, but the service is provided by someone else and open to everyone upon payment. In the COVID-19 context, restrictions related to these two types of transport has generally been limited to the case of different family members travelling in a vehicle, such as setting the maximum number of passengers per vehicle and the use of face coverings or FFP2 masks while travelling.

Public transport on the other hand such as trains, buses, and ferries, was severely affected by the COVID-19 restrictions. Public transport is characterised by a collective use of vehicles, in which many passengers anonymously share an enclosed space while travelling. This is what makes it both an efficient and economical means of transport. This then in turn leads to a high-density use of wagons by many passengers seated or standing within a close distance of one another. This fundamental nature of public transport conflicts with the above-mentioned COVID-19 containment measures. The social distancing rule of 1.5 to 2 meters is irreconcilable to the high-density nature of public transport, while the fall in demand annihilates the economic advantage for those companies providing it. The anonymity also precludes the possibility of contact tracing.

Furthermore, public transport also has the character of a social service to support the mobility of people who do not own or who cannot afford private motorised vehicles. To this end, even under the most stringent movement restrictions, it was essential to keep public transport running in order to support necessary journeys. In the sustainable urban mobility context, public transport is one of the most environmentally-friendly and least carbon-intensive modes of transport, after walking and cycling.

Vienna and Tokyo are both characterised by their high modal shares of public transport. In both cities, public transport supports a large volume of human mobility. When it comes to their respective responses and the ongoing development of said responses to the pandemic, however, the two cities have shown and continue to show different strategies.

The aim of this contribution is to show the impact of COVID-19 on the public transport systems of Vienna and Tokyo. In section one, I present the two cities' public transport systems, their networks and their organisation. In the second section, I analyse and compare the COVID-19 driven responses regarding public transport, and in the third, I look at the long-term effects of the COVID-19 pandemic on the respective public transport systems.

Public transport networks and organisations

Vienna

Network and services

The capital of Austria Vienna had approximately 1.91 million inhabitants as of January 2020, and 1.93 million inhabitants as of January 2022. It covers 415 km2, with 186 km2 (45%) being green space such as agriculture, parks and cemeteries, and forest.[1]

As of the end of 2019, Vienna's urban public transport network consisted of five underground railways (*U-Bahn*) totalling 38 km of track, 28 tram lines covering 225.4 km (if the overlapping part is excluded, 172.0 km), and 131 bus lines making 860.5 km. These are all managed and operated by *Wiener Linien*, a company operating under the auspice of the City of Vienna (although some bus lines are subcontracted to private bus operators).

This primary urban public transport network is supplemented by two other networks. One is the *S-Bahn* (suburban train) and regional train services operated by the passenger division of Austrian Federal Railways (*ÖBB-Personenverkehr*). The so-called *Stammstrecke* (the trunk line) passes through or near the city centre and the *Vorortelinie* (the suburban line) on the western outskirts of the city. Both offer high frequency services comparable to the *U-Bahn*. Additionally, the *Badner Bahn* (*Wiener Lokalbahn*) offers a tram-train service that runs from the city centre to Baden, a spa city located approximately 30 km south of Vienna. Within the city it shares the infrastructure with the *Wiener Linien* trams.

---

[1] Stadt Wien, "Stadtgebiet nach Nutzungsklassen und Bezirken 2022."

In addition to these daytime services, night buses (*Nightlines*) are provided on a daily basis with 30-minute intervals throughout the night after the last daytime service around midnight until the first daytime service around 5:00 am. Since 2010, night underground services have also been provided on Friday and Saturday nights, as well as the nights before public holidays with 15-minute intervals.

Users

In 2019, underground railways carried 459.8 million passengers, tramways carried 304.8 million passengers, and buses carried 196.1 million passengers – in total 960.7 million passengers for the whole year or 2,63 million passengers per day.[2] Approximately 852,000 annual travel passes valid for the city were sold in 2019.[3]

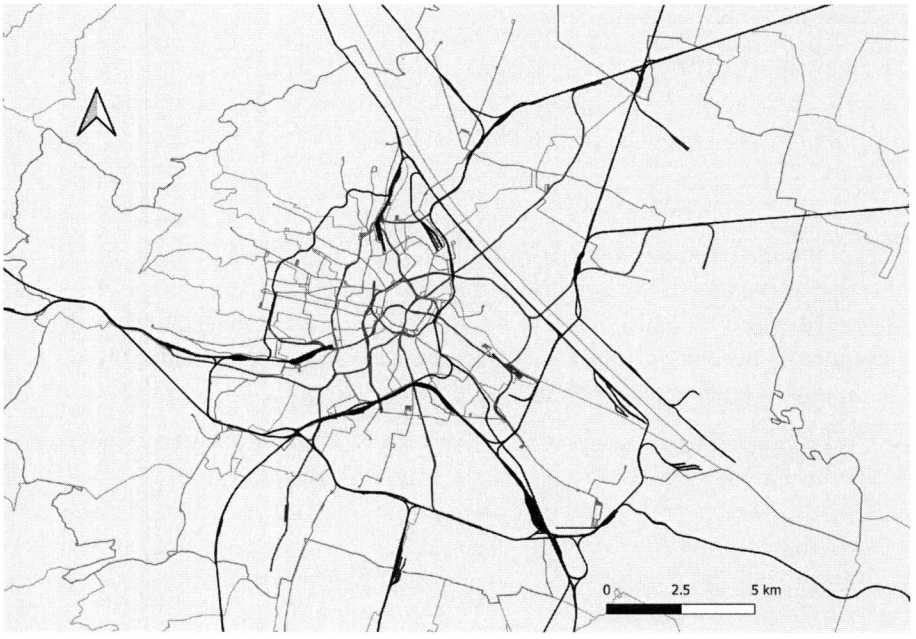

Fig.1: Vienna's rail, underground and tramway network
(Illustration: Takeru Shibayama)

---

[2] Wiener Linien, "Zahlen & Fakten Betriebsangaben 2019."
[3] Ibid.

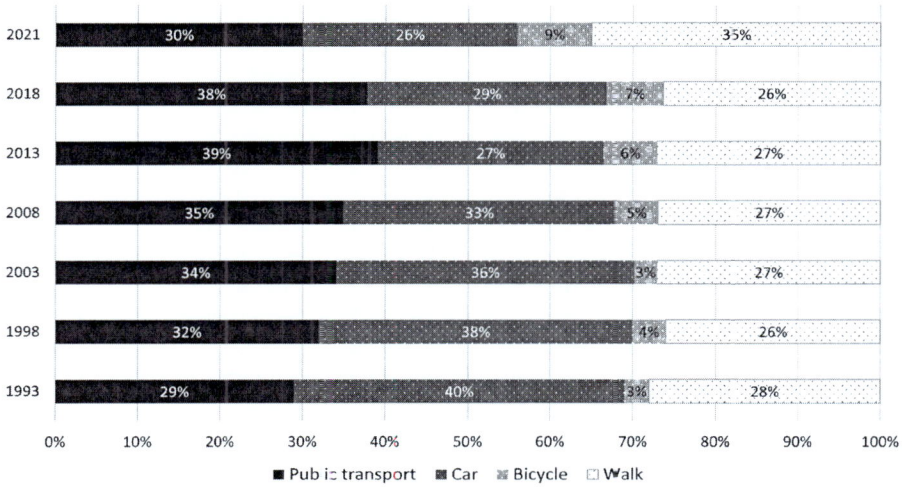

Fig. 2: Modal share, Vienna (Illustration: Takeru Shibayama)

Organisations

Both *Wiener Linien* and the *Badner Bahn* are publicly owned enterprises controlled indirectly by the City of Vienna. The Austrian Federal Railway (*ÖBB*) is fully owned by the Federal Government. As such, all primary public transport operators in Vienna are public sector companies.

Following both EU and national regulations these public transport services fall under the auspices of the corresponding competent authorities. The City of Vienna is the competent authority for the *Wiener Linien* services, while the Federal Government is the competent authority for the regional train network providing the national minimal service according to the service level of 1999/2000 timetables as stipulated by the Public Transport Act (*Öffentlicher Personennah- und Regionalverkehrsgesetz 1999 - ÖPNRV-G 1999*). Additional regional rail services, as well as the *Badner Bahn* and regional bus services are run under the auspices of the the VOR (*Verkehrsverbund Ost-Region*). Providing public transport services to the greater Vienna region, *VOR* is the competent regional public transport authority jointly established by the City of Vienna along with the Federal States of Lower Austria and Burgenland. *VOR* is responsible for the coordination and tariff integration of public transport.

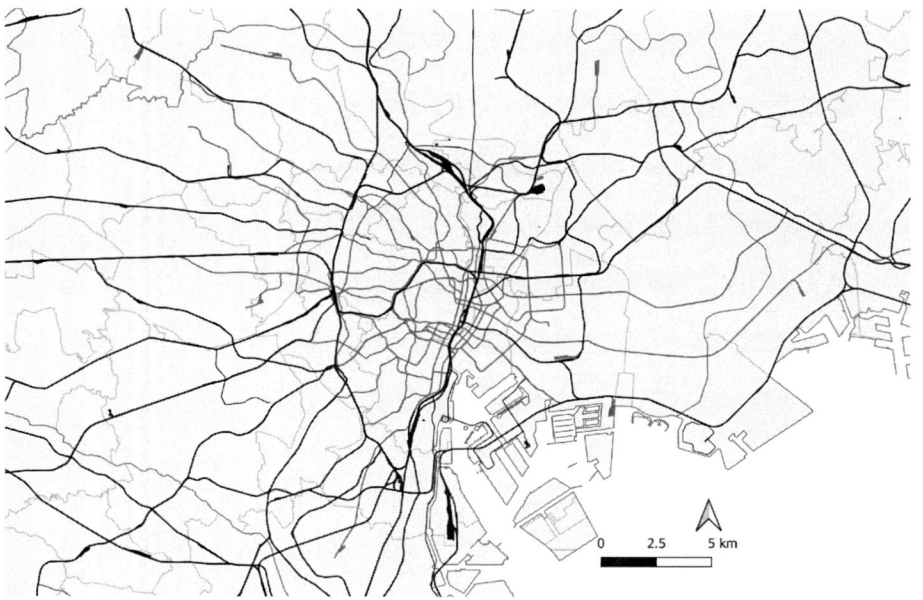

Fig. 3: Railway network, Central Tokyo (Illustration: Takeru Shibayama)

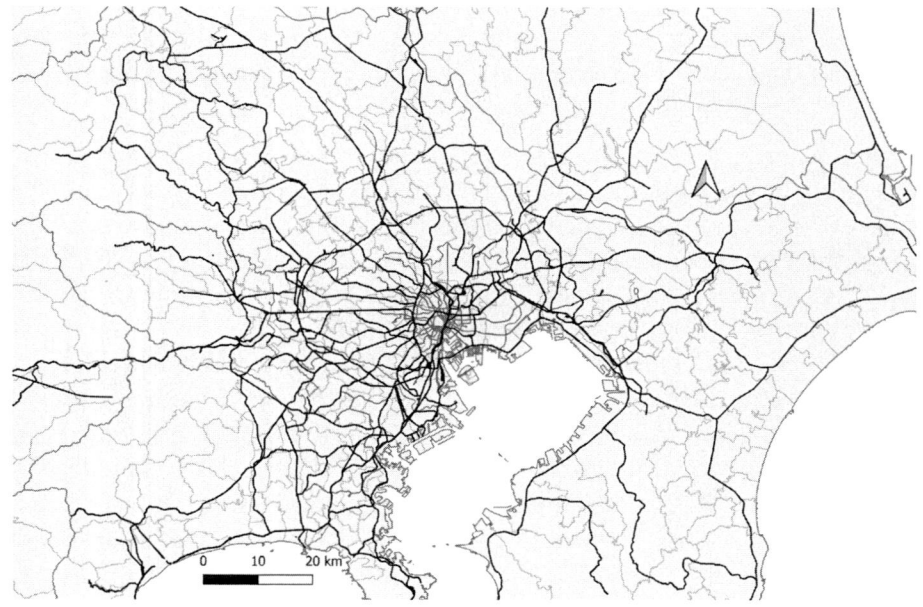

Fig. 4: Railway network, Greater Tokyo Area (Illustration: Takeru Shibayama)

Tokyo

Network

"Tokyo" is an extensive area and there are several different definitions in terms of its territoriality. The smallest definition is the area covered by the Special Wards of Tokyo (*Tokubetsu-ku*), an area of 627.51 km2 with approximately 9.78 million inhabitants, making c. a. 15,500 inhabitants per km2 .The area of the Tokyo Metropolitan Government covers the Special Wards and a further 30 municipalities west of the Special Wards, with 14 million inhabitants. The Greater Tokyo Area consists of a much wider area including parts of neighboring prefectures and is comparable to a Functional Urban Area as defined by the OECD and the EU. According to the OECD, the Tokyo Metropolitan Area has 35.7 million inhabitants and stretches over several prefectures surrounding it[4].

Reflecting its size, Tokyo's public transport network is extensive with 2,705 km of railway network and 1,510 stations as of 2015[5], complemented by feeder bus services as well as other modes of public transport such as the AGT and monorails. The urban railway network of *JR East* and eight other private railway companies, namely *Keikyu, Keio, Keisei, Odakyu, Sagami (Sotetsu), Seibu, Tobu,* and *Tokyu Railways* compose the backbone of the network, supplemented by many smaller private railway companies. The *Tokyo Metro* operates nine lines in the centre of Tokyo, while *Toei* Subway, which is operated by the Tokyo Metropolitan Government, also operates four subway lines. The outer centres of Tokyo, such as Yokohama and Chiba, also have underground railway services or the AGT. Public-private joint ventures are also often used to operate relatively new railway lines in the suburbs and outskirts of Tokyo, especially newer railway lines built after the 1990s.

This trunk railway network is complemented by feeder bus services. While *JR East* and *Tokyo Metro* does not offer bus services, the eight major private railway companies and the *Toei* operate their bus services in the area where they operate railway services. Further independent bus operators exist, complementing these companies.

---

[4] OECD, "Maskenpflicht in Handel und Öffis fällt ab Juni, Wien geht strengeren Weg."
[5] Koutsu-Seisaku-Shingikai, "Tokyo-ken-ni-okeru Kongo-no Toshi-tetsudo-no Arikata-ni-tsuite." (The report is only published every 15 years, so the 2014 figures are the most recent. However, it is assumed that these did not change significantly until shortly before the pandemic.).

Users

According to a report submitted to MLIT in 2014[6], Tokyo's urban railway system carries approximately 22.5 million passengers per day.

Figure 5 is a summary of modal share in the Greater Tokyo Area, as well as the central 23 wards of Tokyo (Central Tokyo) based on the results of Person-Trip Surveys which take place every 10 years. What is remarkable is the very high share of railways in the centre – above 50 % – as well as the high share of bicycles and walking. In the Greater Tokyo Area, automobiles have some roles comparable to that of Vienna, but in Central Tokyo, it is one of the least chosen modes. Both in the city centre and in the Greater Tokyo Area, active modes (walking and cycling together) have approximately one third of the modal share. As such, Tokyo's transport system is extremely dependent on public transport and active modes. The very high share of public transport in the central 23 words is the primary driver of the high modal share of public transport in the Greater Tokyo Area as a whole.

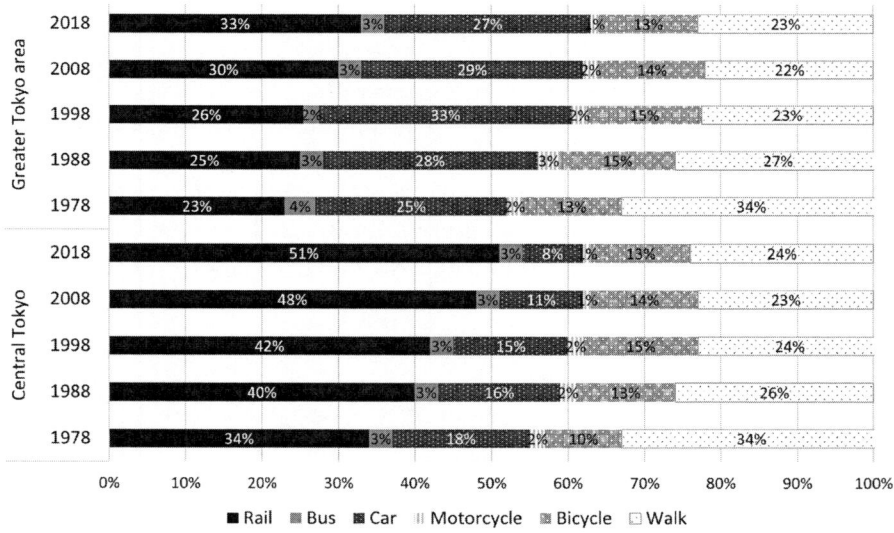

Fig. 5: Modal share: Greater Tokyo Area and Central Tokyo, 23 Wards
(Illustration: Takeru Shibayama)

---

[6] Ibid.

Organisations

Tokyo's public transport network is characterised by being primarily organised and run by the private sector including the aforementioned *JR East* and the major private railways. The underground railways, however, are primarily operated by public sector institutions, such as the *Tokyo Metro*, the *Toei*, and the *Yokohama City Transportation Bureau*. It is worth noting that *Tokyo Metro* is a corporation under private law but is owned by the National and Tokyo Metropolitan Governments, and thus has a public character. Nevertheless, all these public sector enterprises operating public transport are obliged to operate on a financially self-sustaining basis, as stipulated in the Local Public Enterprise Act (*Chiho-Kouei-Kigyou-Hou*). Under this Act, the principle of private corporate accounting is also applied to public enterprises operating public transport services. The same principle applies to public-private joint ventures, too. As such, Tokyo's public transport system is organised principally as a private sector business, no matter the nature of the legal status of each given enterprise.

Buses are operated on a similar principle to that of the railway. The aforementioned eight major private railway companies all have subsidiaries operating buses, while other operators only offer bus services. The Tokyo Metropolitan Government, as well as the *Kawasaki* and *Yokohama City Transportation Bureaus* provide bus services within their jurisdictions. In total, 77 bus operators operate in the Greater Tokyo Area.

First public transport responses to COVID-19

Vienna

The very first case of COVID-19 in Austria was registered on 25 February 2020 in Innsbruck. Parallel to the declaration of a pandemic by the WHO on 11 March 2020, Austria introduced several measures such as restrictions on international travel, the cancellation of events (10 March 2020), the closure of schools and universities (11 March 2020), and the closure of retail stores deemed non-essential (16 March 2020).

The Federal Government introduced a nationwide lockdown on 16th March 2020. Starting on this day, it was forbidden to leave home except for the following reasons: avoiding immediate danger, helping people in need of support (e.g., family care), carrying out essential purchases such as groceries, and occupation-relevant purposes ("essential" workers). Walking or fitness activities such as cycling or jogging either alone or with members of household was also allowed[7]. Starting on 20 March 2020, wherever possible people were recommended to work from home[8].

This first general lockdown was lifted on 1 May 2020. In response to later waves, lockdowns were repeatedly enforced in Vienna for a total of five times so far as summarised below.

#	Type	Duration
1	National	**16 March 2020 to 1 May 2020**, with stepwise reopening from 14 April
2	National	**17 November 2020 – 6 December 2020**, with "lockdown light" between 3 November 2020 to 16 November 2020 and 7 December 2020 to 23 December 2020 when a curfew was in place between 8pm and 6am.
3	National	**26 December 2020 to 7 February 2021**, then "lockdown light" starting on 8 February
4	Regional	**1 April to 2 May 2021**, *East-Region Lockdown* in Vienna, Lower Austria and Burgenland (Burgenland until 19 April), then "lockdown light" until 30 June 2022.
5	National	**22 November 2021 to 19 December 2021** in Vienna only, with a "lockdown for the non-vaccinated" before, after and during this period nationwide.

Table 1: Summary of COVID-19 lockdowns in Vienna

Already before the first lockdown, *Wiener Linien* reported a reduction in passenger numbers of more than 20 % as of 13 March 2020. After the announcement of the lockdown, a sudden drop in passenger numbers was reported. On 16 March 2020, *Wiener Linien* reported a reduction of up to 40 %[9], a further reduction of up to 60 % on 17 March 2020[10], and finally up to 80 % on 20 March 2020[11]. Similarly, the Federal Railway *ÖBB* reported a 70 % reduction of passenger numbers on 17 March 2020[12] on a nationwide scale. Responding to the reduced demand, *Wiener Linien* adjusted its weekday public transport services to the school holiday timetable on 18 March 2020, followed by a further adjustment to the Saturday timetable starting on 23 March 202[13]. Night-time services were suspended on 20 March 2020[14]. As such, and in synchronisation with the lockdown, Vienna's public transport service was reduced quickly using existing timetables in response to the fall in demand.

---

[7] Bundeskanzleramt, "Bundesgesetzblatt BGBl II Nr. 98/2020."
[8] Bundeskanzleramt, "Bundesgesetzblatt BGBl II Nr. 108/2020."
[9] Vienna Online, "Coronavirus: Bis zu 40 Prozent weniger Fahrgäste bei den Wiener Linien."
[10] Vienna Online, "Wiener Linien vermelden 60 Prozent weniger Fahrgäste wegen Coronakrise."
[11] Vienna Online, "80 Prozent weniger Fahrgäste: Wiener Linien passen Fahrplan an."
[12] Vienna Online, "Wiener Linien vermelden 60 Prozent weniger Fahrgäste wegen Coronakrise."
[13] Vienna Online, "80 Prozent weniger Fahrgäste: Wiener Linien passen Fahrplan an."
[14] Vienna Online, "Coronavirus: Wiener Linien passen Fahrplan an."

A series of on-board protection measures were introduced, too[15]. On 16 March 2020, the first entrance door and the seating near the driver in both buses and older tramways were closed for passengers[16]. Button-operated doors were operated automatically[17]. As of 14 April, despite lockdown measures being somewhat eased at this time, it became mandatory to wear a face covering on public transport. At the beginning, any kind of face covering that covered the mouth and nose was accepted, but on 25 January 2021 the mandatory use of an FFP2 mask came into force. While the nationwide regulation of wearing face coverings – either FFP2 or otherwise – on public transport was lifted on 1 July 2022, the FFP2 regulation continues in Vienna up to the time of writing (September 2022).[18]

An interesting measure introduced during the first lockdown in Vienna was the distribution of taxi vouchers equivalent to EUR 50 for elderly people aged over 65. This measure was introduced by the City of Vienna. Approximately 300,000 elderly people were able to profit from this. The city justified this as the use of taxis reduced the risk of infection compared to public transport, where possible contact to other people could occur.[19] Furthermore, the City of Vienna eliminated the payable parking zones in the city and reduced the price of car parks[20].

Tokyo

The very first case of a COVID-19 infection in Japan was registered as early as 16 January 2020, just a few weeks after the first case was reported in late December 2019 in Wuhan, China. An individual who had stayed in Wuhan and lived in Kanagawa, near Tokyo, was the first person to be diagnosed with COVID-19. On 4 February 2020, 10 positive cases were detected aboard the cruise ship *Diamond Princess*, which had docked at Yokohama on the previous day. On 13 February 2020, the first COVID-19 fatality was reported. As such, the virus reached Japan very quickly. This did not, however, lead to strong containment measures at this time (1st Wave).

The situation changed starting in late March 2020, when a rapid increase in positive cases was reported almost simultaneously to those being reported

---

[15] Austria introduced the mandatory use of face masks relatively early in Europe: in retails, it was made mandatory as early as the end of March 2020.
[16] Vienna Online, "Wiener Linien vermelden 60 Prozent weniger Fahrgäste wegen Coronakrise."
[17] Vienna Online, "80 Prozent weniger Fahrgäste: Wiener Linien passen Fahrplan an."
[18] Springer, "Maskenpflicht in Handel und Öffis fällt ab Juni, Wien geht strengeren Weg."
[19] RND, "Coronavirus-Krise: Stadt Wien spendiert Senioren freie Taxi-Fahrten."
[20] Gebhard, "Wiener Kurzparkzonen ab Dienstag aufgehoben."

in Europe and North America. On 7 April 2020, an Epidemic Emergency was declared in the Tokyo Metropolitan Area (Tokyo, Saitama, Chiba, and Kanagawa), Osaka, Hyogo and Fukuoka prefectures. On 16 April 2020, this was extended to the rest of the country. This continued until 25 May 2020 in the Tokyo Metropolitan Area. Differently from lockdowns, during the Epidemic Emergency in Japan, it was not prohibited to carry out activities outside of one's home. Nevertheless, staying at home was strongly recommended, with clear guidance from all levels of government.

Tokyo's public transport is characterised by its very intensive nature, leading to overcrowded rail services during peak hours. Reflecting this, the country showed a very high level of interest in whether or not public transport was a high-risk environment for COVID-19 infections, as seen, for example, in various media articles. In February 2020, the national epidemiology committee published its preliminary finding that public transport did not fulfill the three conditions that lead to COVID-19 clusters, later known as the 3Cs – Closed Spaces, Crowded Places, and Close-contact Settings. The committee argued that public transport does not fulfill the Close-contact Settings, where oral communication among people take place. Thus, compared to other conditions fulfilling the 3Cs, public transport is less likely to become the place for cluster building.

Since the beginning of the pandemic, the Ministry of Land, Infrastructure, Transport and Tourism (MLIT) has reviewed the changes in passenger volumes monthly with questionnaires to operators. According to their May 2020 report, among the major private railways (including the eight from Tokyo, as well as ones from the region of Kansai and from the city of Fukuoka), 86 % experienced a reduction of 50–70 % in passenger volumes, and 14 % experienced a reduction of more than 70 % in passenger volumes[21] compared to the same month in the previous year.

Another characteristic of Japan is that the major public transport operators mentioned above are among Designated Institutions of a Public Nature nominated by the Office for Pandemic Influenza and New Infectious Disease Preparedness and Response at the national Cabinet Secretariat. Such designated institutions include medical facilities and pharmaceutical companies, energy companies, telecommunication companies and public transport and logistics companies. The designation is stipulated by Article 2, Paragraph 7 of the national *Act on Special Measures against Pandemic Influenza and New Infectious*

---

[21] MLIT, "Shingata-Koronauirusu-Kansensho-ni-tomonau Kankei-Gyoukai-no Eikyo-ni-tsuite."

Diseases Preparedness and Response, which was promulgated in 2012[22] and applied to COVID-19. In article 53, this Act stipulates that the designated institutions are required to take any measures to enable the continued transport of passengers and goods in case of an epidemic emergency. The major public transport operators in Tokyo including *JR East* and the eight major private railways are all designated here at the national level. Other railway operators are designated in the prefectures where they operate. Within this legal framework, each railway operator was required to draw up a contingency plan in case of an epidemic, such as the one published by *JR East*[23], and to continue to provide transport services so that passenger transport is appropriately ensured during epidemics.

With this background, even though service is based on private-sector financing, and despite the dramatic reduction in passenger volume, Japan's public transport has continued to operate normally during the 1st stage of the COVID-19 pandemic.

Month 2020	No impact	0 to -10%	-10 to -20%	-20 to -30%	-30 to -50%	-50 to -70%	Less than -70%
February	8	8	0	0	0	0	0
March	0	0	2	13	1	0	0
April	0	0	0	0	13	3	0
May	0	0	0	0	14	2	0
June	0	0	0	11	5	0	0
July	0	0	0	12	4	0	0
August	0	0	0	14	2	0	0
September	0	0	0	7	9	0	0
October	0	0	1	14	1	0	0
November	0	0	4	11	1	0	0
December	0	0	3	12	1	0	0

Table 2: Reduction of passenger volumes among 16 major private railway operators in 2020, Tokyo (number of operators in the range of reduction by month, table based on the report by MLIT as of 30 April 2020[24] and as of 31 December 2020[25])

It is also worth noting that, reflecting the 2012 Act, a research institute directly under MLIT carried out a survey to public transport operators and

---

[22] e-gov, "Shingata-Infruenza-tou Taisaku Tokubetsu-sochi-hou."
[23] JR East, "Shingata-Infuruenza-tou Taisaku-Gyoumu-Keikaku Youshi."
[24] Ibid., 7.
[25] MLIT, "Shingata-Koronauirusu-Kansensho-ni-tomonau Kankei-Gyoukai-no Eikyo-ni-tsuite."

held an expert panel discussion, which was published in 2015[26]. In this report, five measures were discussed, including the advocation of "cough etiquette" on board and at stations (e. g., cover mouth when coughing), the use of non-woven face masks, the prohibition of the use of public transport by infected passengers, the disinfection of wagons and station facilities, and recommendations of frequent hand washing and disinfections. In response to COVID-19, MLIT already requested railway operators on 31 January 2020, as well as on 24 February 2020 to take these protection measures onboard and at stations. MLIT also requested them to closely monitor the health conditions of staff at the same time. Similar requests were made to the bus operators around the same time, too[27].

Comparison

Responding to both the drop in demand and the national lockdown public transport services in Vienna were adjusted to the school holiday and weekend timetables beginning in March 2020.

Protection measures were more rule-based, such as the prohibition of leaving one's home (albeit with some exceptions), and the mandatory use of first face coverings and then later FFP2 masks on public transport. It is notable that the City of Vienna implemented some measures favouring the use of private vehicles.

After the early detection of the virus in Japan, pre-defined procedures and prevention measures for public transport put into place during the H1N1 influenza outbreak in 2009 guided the authorities and operators in their response.

As a result, public transport services were initially maintained at pre-pandemic levels despite the drastic fall in passenger volume while at the same time prevention measures and information about the risk of infection were communicated to passengers well before the announcement of an Epidemic Emergency.

This demonstrates that the public transport sector in Japan shows a high degree of preparedness for an epidemic of respiratory diseases. Contrary to Vienna, the Epidemic Emergency was on a recommendation only basis, and as such users of public transport were able to make their own decision as to whether they would follow the said recommendations.

---

[26] Hase et al., "Research onto Measures for Public Transport Addressing Epidemic of Novel Influenza."
[27] MLIT, "Kokudo-Koutsu-Sho-ni-okeru Shingata-Koronauirusu-Kansensho-heno Taiou-joukyou."

Mid- to long-term changes of public transport systems

Vienna

After the first lockdown was lifted on 1 May 2020, on 11 May 2020, the *U-Bahn* services were put back to the pre-COVID service level, and at the same time, shorter interval on a part of the line U6 was implemented as planned before[28]. On 18 May 2020, the tram and bus services were put back to the normal pre-COVID service levels. The night-time bus service was put back, too, while the night-time underground services in Vienna was suspended until June 2021[29]. As such, except for night-time underground service, the public transport services in Vienna were put back to the pre-COVID level quickly soon after the first lockdown was lifted.

A wide range of improvements to public transport services have taken place in Austria in recent times and indeed several are still ongoing. Already in May 2020, the Federal Government announced an extra EUR 300 million investment in public transport in the context of supporting the national economy: half of it for the improvement of infrastructure in particular regional railways, and the rest to increase service levels[30]. The European Commission also set up a large funding scheme named *NextGen EU* to help Member States recover from the pandemic. Under this scheme, measures in the two specific areas of *green transition* and *digital transition* are to be given preference. In Austria, under the theme of *green transition*, EUR 843 million is foreseen in the domain of *sustainable mobility with zero-emission transport*, and an additional EUR 543 million is foreseen as *investment in an electrified trans-European railway network*. This is coupled with a tax reform in 2022 which introduced a tax on CO_2 emissions. A so-called climate bonus *(Klimabonus)* is being paid out to individuals to compensate for additional energy costs with the exact amount depending on regional factors, including the quality and availability of local public transport.[31]

Among ticketing offers, the highlight is the introduction of a *Klimaticket* (Climate Ticket), another Federal Government measure enabling unlimited travel on all public transport throughout the whole of Austria for EUR 1,065 per year or for a specific region or combination of regions for a lesser amount, like the existing Annual Travel Pass *(Jahreskarte)* for Vienna, and as well as the newly-introduced regional version covering the whole VOR area (the federal

---

[28] Fabry, Clemens, "Weiterhin keine Nacht-U-Bahn in Wien."
[29] Vienna Online, "Nacht-U-Bahn fährt in Wien wieder."
[30] ORF, "300 Mio. Euro mehr für öffentlichen Verkehr."
[31] European Commission, "Austria's Recovery and Resilience Plan."

states of Vienna, Lower Austria and Burgenland) for EUR 915 per year. The nationwide version started on 26 October 2021. As of July 2022, 185,809 nationwide *Klimatickets* had been sold, among which 58,709 (31.6%) were sold in Vienna[32]. This is much higher in comparison to the proportion of the population of Vienna to the total Austrian population (21.7%), implying that public transport users in Vienna benefit from the *Klimaticket* more than those in other federal states.

Tokyo

As briefly mentioned before, Japan did not implement a stringent lockdown comparable to many Western countries. Rather, under the national Epidemic Emergency, crossing prefectural borders was discouraged, and the gastronomy sector, particularly where alcohol was served, was encouraged to close early at 8:00pm with the government providing subsidies to those venues which followed this recommendation.

Additionally, while there was no obligation to stay at home, many companies voluntarily introduced work-from-home schemes.

Even after such recommendations were discontinued, the number of people going out in the evening in Tokyo remained lower than pre-pandemic. The data collected by Agoop for the time period on 6 Oct 2022, more than two years after the beginning of the pandemic, based on mobile phone locations and visualised by NHK, a national TV sender, show that the number of people actively out in the centre of Tokyo between 6:00–9:00 pm had fallen between 5 to 30% compared to the weekday average of the pre-pandemic period of 18 January – 24 February 2020. A similar tendency was shown in the nightlife districts of Shinjuku and Shibuya, as well as other sub-centres such as Kichijoji between 9:00pm and midnight.[33] For example, as of 6 October 2022 between 9:00pm and midnight the Kabukicho neighbourhood of Shinjuku registered 19.6% fewer people, and Shibuya nightlife district registered 16.5% fewer people compared to the weekday average of the same time period between 18 January and 14 February 2020 before the pandemic was declared.

In the same comparison between pre-pandemic average and the data on 6 October 2022- but during the day, the reduction in the number of people in the office district in the centre of Tokyo is also remarkable, with around 30% fewer people observed throughout the day in the districts of Shinagawa, Shimbasi

---

[32] BMK, "Zahlen, Daten, Fakten zu den Klimatickets."
[33] NHK, "Machino-hitode-ha? Zenkoku 18-chiten Gurafu."

and Yaesu. This is also reflected in the peak-hour congestion rate on commuter railways, an indicator commonly used in Japan to compare the ratio of passengers passing though pre-defined sample cross-sections to the total nominal capacity provided through the same cross-sections. Until 2019, this rate was constant at around 165 % among the 31 sample cross-sections within the Tokyo Metropolitan Area. In 2020, it dropped to 107 %, remaining relatively stable in 2021 at 108 %. Through these 31 sample cross-sections, peak-hour passenger volume stayed around 1.6 million between 2013–2020 and then fell abruptly to around 1.06 million with no change in 2021. As such, the morning peak-hour is much eased, the number of peak-hour commuters having decreased radically.

The reduction in passenger volume can be seen in the statistics, too. Figure 6 is an overview of the passenger-kilometers transported by the eight major private railways, *Tokyo Metro, Toei Subway*, and a selection of *JR lines* during the fiscal years of 2019 and 2020 (both starting in April and ending in March). It can be seen that the largest relative drop occurred on the *Keisei* line. This is probably because of the fall in demand for international air travel, the *Keisei* line being the rail connection for Narita Airport, the primary airport for international air traffic.

A significant fall in passenger volume can also be seen on the *JR Yamanote* Line, which is the ring railway line. Also on the *Odakyu, Keio* and *Tokyu* railways. These are the lines characterised by relatively long travel distances from their respective terminus stations of Shinjuku (*Odakyu* and *Keio*) and Shibuya (*Tokyu*), and also by relatively high-income commuters and thus presumably a higher share of office workers living along the routes. A similar fall in passenger volume can also be observed for the *Chuo* line (one of the *JR* lines), this line having a similar character. The higher drop in passenger-kilometers transported on these aforementioned lines clearly demonstrates a reduction in long-distance commuting due to large numbers of office workers moving to a work-from-home model.

It can be seen then that there were notable reductions in the number of people out of their homes both in the typical office areas, as well as in the nightlife districts. This tendency continues up to the time of writing, after more than 30 months since the beginning of the COVID-19 pandemic. The clear implication is that the work-from-home model, which was primarily introduced by many offices as a response to COVID-19, has become well established in Tokyo as a common practice. As a result, the classic after-work *nomikai* (drinking session) culture, which was common among workplace colleagues[34], has shrunk in line with the adoption of this new model. The rapid diffusion of work-from-home is

---

[34] INTAGE Inc., "Kaisha-gaeri-ni Nomikai Shitemasuka?"

particularly understandable in the Tokyo context, with much longer commutes compared to many other cities, and where people were forced to travel in overcrowded commuter trains.

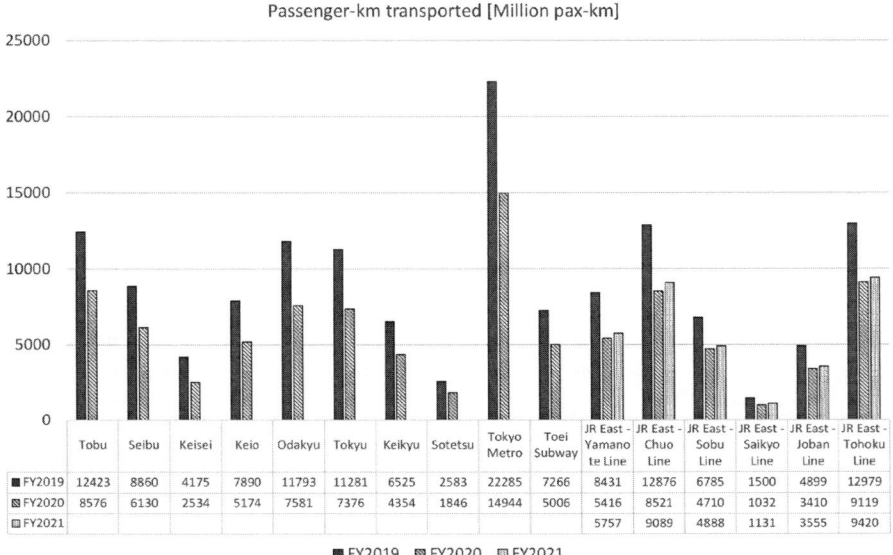

Fig. 6: Passenger-km transported by 8 Major private railways, Tokyo Metro, Toei subway and a selection of JR Lines (Illustration: Takeru Shibayama)

In response to this change in lifestyle, the public transport operators have adjusted their timetables, especially in the late evening hours after 9:00pm. After the declaration of the pandemic in March 2020, many operators adjusted their regular timetables by bringing the last service forward to an earlier time. A symbolically significant decision was also taken to cancel the night-time bus service from Shibuya to the western residential districts. The so-called *Midnight Arrow* was suspended in the early phase of the pandemic, and then decided not to resume in July 2022[35]. Established in the late 1980s, this night bus service was a product of the Bubble Economy era. Its closure meant the disappearance of one of the last living vestiges of this economic heyday. Later on, some daytime services in the city centre were also reduced, for example

---

[35] Tokyu Bus Corporation, "Shinya-Kyuko-Basu oyobi Tsukin-Kosoku-Basu Haishi-no Oshirase. "

in the August 2022 timetable adjustment of the *Tokyo Metro* in response to reduced demand[36]. Table 3 is a summary of the five major stations in Tokyo, showing the timetable before and after the adjustment: depending on the line, the last train was brought forward by up to 35 minutes.

Station	Operator	Direction	Last train as of March 2017	Last train as of September 2022
Tokyo	JR East	Yamanote Line, Clockwise to Shinagawa	1:03	0:46
		Yamanote Line, Counterclockwise to Ikebukuro	0:37	0:38
		Chuo Line westbound to Mitaka	0:35	0:05
		Chuo Line westbound to Takao	0:20	23:45
Ueno		Joban Line (Rapid) to Matsudo	0:51	0:33
Shinjuku	Odakyu	To Sagami-Ohno	0:38	0:15
	Keio	To Keio-Hachioji	0:33	0:18
Shibuya	Tokyu	Toyoko Line via Yokohama to Motomachi-Chukagai	0:07	23:38
		Den-en-toshi Line to Chuo-Rinkan	0:15	23:52
Ikebukuro	Seibu	Ikebukuro Line to Hanno (Semi-Express)	0:08	23:52
	Tobu	Tojo Line to Shinrin-Koen	0:02	0:02

Table 3: Comparison of the last public transport services at major stations in Tokyo between 2017 and 2022

Comparison

In Vienna, the impact on the public transport system in the long run has been relatively small. While demand does not yet seem to have returned to previous highs, the service level has returned to the pre-pandemic timetables, or in some cases even improved. With the increased awareness of climate issues both Vienna's public transport system in particular, and Austria's public transport system in general, have gained much political leverage in recent times – given their environmentally-friendly and low-energy nature. This can be interpreted as a reflection of the character of the public sector organisation public transport in Austria, which is embedded in a wider socio-economic context.

In contrast, in the long-run, Tokyo's public transport has seen more changes. The establishment of work-from-home practices has clearly benefited and continues to benefit many office workers otherwise faced with long commuting hours. This has led to a decrease in the number of commuters. Similarly, the pandemic has impacted night life culture to a large extent, also leading to a

---

[36] Tokyo Metro Co. Ltd., "News Release," 22–38.

reduction in passenger volume during the evening and night-time hours. At the time of writing, this is around 30%, although some rebound in the near future cannot be excluded. The reduction of passengers has led to a reduction in late evening and night-time public transport services, and also some daytime services. This is an understandable reaction from a public transport system that largely functions as a private business model, whereby reduced demand leads to lower profit margins. This is already very visible with public transport in rural areas and small cities[37], while the same issue is starting to affect large cities including Tokyo. An institutional reform of the public transport sector has been put on the agenda among leading experts in the country, and potentially the COVID-19 pandemic will be understood as the trigger for future institutional reform.

Discussion and Conclusion

Prior to the COVID-19 pandemic, people's travel behaviour around both Vienna's and Tokyo's public transport networks showed similar patterns. The modal shares of public transport were both approximately one-third of all journeys. The initial response to COVID-19 showed a clear difference in that Vienna's accompanied the national lockdown on an ad-hoc rule-based measure, while Tokyo's response can be interpreted as an exercise of prepared epidemic responses based on previous learning from H1N1.

Vienna's public transport has retained the organisation and strategy it had before the COVID-19 pandemic. Its position at the core of the response to the climate crisis in terms of being an environmentally-friendly and low-energy form of transport, along with walking and cycling, has been retained, and indeed strengthened with clear political pushes from different levels of government, as well as help from the European COVID-19 recovery fund. Within the city's actual mobility masterplan *STEP 2025 - Mobility*, Vienna has set a strategic goal of bringing up the modal share of active modes and public transport to 80% and bringing down that of automobiles to 20% by 2025[38]. The Austrian Federal Government also has a general goal of climate neutrality by 2040[39].

---

[37] Chiiki-Koukyou-Koutsu Sogo-Kenkyuusho, "Dai-4-kai Koukyou-koutsu Keiei-jittai Chousa Houkokusho."

[38] Vienna City Administration Municipal Dept. 18, STEP 2025 Thematic Concept - Urban Mobility Plan Vienna.

[39] Bundeskanzleramt, "Aus Verantwortung für Österreich: Regierungsprogramm 2020–2024."

As such, prioritising public transport is embedded in long-term sustainability goals.

Tokyo, however, has experienced a reduction in public transport services triggered by the pandemic. A clear upcoming challenge is to find a path back to pre-pandemic levels as a part of the overall urban infrastructure. Until now, public transport's response in Tokyo is largely limited to passive adjustments of timetables in attempts to cover operational costs with reduced travel demand. If the new income-expense balance of public transport operators remains firm for a longer period, a new organisational and institutional structure may be needed, such as involvement of public-sector financing for operation. This may well lead to significant institutional reform.

It is also worth noting that the pre-pandemic high modal share of public transport was mainly driven by the high modal share in the city centre of Tokyo. The primary users supporting this were commuters who have since shifted to working from home – at least partially – and this trend is expected to continue beyond the pandemic. This may lead to a shift of activity centres of previous rail commuters to the outskirts of Tokyo, where the modal share of automobile is relatively high. Thus, the altered working style and lifestyle hold a reasonable risk of a potential shift of travel modes towards an increased use of private motorised forms of transport, which in the wider context of climate issues should be avoided. The current weakness of Tokyo is that it still lacks a strategic mobility masterplan[40] comparable to Europe's *Sustainable Urban Mobility Plans*. An awareness of the changes in both commuter and lifestyle choices described above and resulting from COVID-19 should serve as a good starting point for developing such a plan.

Bibliography

Technologie, Innovation). "Zahlen, Daten, Fakten zu den Klimatickets." Accessed October 7, 2022. www.bmk.gv.at//themen//mobilitaet//1-2-3-ticket//fakten.htm.

Bundeskanzleramt. "Aus Verantwortung Für Österreich: Regierungsprogramm 2020–2024." www.dieneuevolkspartei.at/Download/Regierungsprogramm_2020.pdf.

Bundeskanzleramt. "Bundesgesetzblatt BGBl II Nr. 108/2020."

Bundeskanzleramt. "Bundesgesetzblatt BGBl II Nr. 98/2020." www.ris.bka.gv.at/Dokumente/BgblAuth/BGBLA_2020_II_98/BGBLA_2020_II_98.pdfsig.

---

[40] Shibayama, "Competence Distribution and Policy Implementation Efficiency Towards Sustainable Urban Transport: A Comparative Study."

Chiiki-Koukyou-Koutsu Sogo-Kenkyuusho. "Dai-4-kai Koukyou-koutsu Keiei-jittai Chousa Houkokusho." *The Research Institute of Local Public Transport*, 2022. URL: https://ryobi.gr.jp/wp-content/uploads/2022/08/4thchikoken.pdf.

e-gov. "Shingata-Infruenza-Tou Taisaku Tokubetsu-Sochi-Hou." Accessed October 5, 2022. https://elaws.e-gov.go.jp/document?lawid=424AC0000000031_20220617_504AC0000000068.

European Commission. "Austria's Recovery and Resilience Plan." Accessed October 7, 2022. https://ec.europa.eu/info/business-economy-euro/recovery-coronavirus/recovery-and-resilience-facility/austrias-recovery-and-resilience-plan_en.

Fabry, Clemens. "Weiterhin keine Nacht-U-Bahn in Wien." *Die Presse*, May 4, 2020. www.diepresse.com/5808870/weiterhin-keine-nacht-u-bahn-in-wien.

Gebhard, Josef. "Wiener Kurzparkzonen ab Dienstag Aufgehoben." *Der Kurier*, March 16, 2020. https://kurier.at/chronik/wien/coronavirus-wiener-kurzparkzonen-ab-dienstag-aufgehoben/400782251.

Hase, T., S. Nakao, K. Kikuchi, and K. Kato. "Research into Measures for Public Transport Addressing Epidemic of Novel Influenza." *PRI Review* 55 (2015): 34–47. www.mlit.go.jp/pri/kikanshi/pdf/pri_review_55.pdf.

INTAGE Inc. "Kaisha-gaeri-ni Nomikai Shitemasuka?" Accessed October 7, 2022. https://gallery.intage.co.jp/nomikai2017/.

Jorudan Co. L. "Jorudan." Accessed October 5, 2022. www.jorudan.co.jp.

JR East. "Shingata-Infuruenza-tou Taisaku-Gyoumu-Keikaku Youshi" www.jreast.co.jp/company/pdf/influenza_gyoumukeikaku.pdf.

JTB. *JTB Jikokuhyou 2017-3*. Tokyo: JTB Publishing, 2017.

Koutsu-Seisaku-Shingikai. "Tokyo-ken-ni-okeru Kongo-no Toshi-tetsudo-no Arikata-ni-tsuite." www.mlit.go.jp/common/001138591.pdf.

MLIT. "Kokudo-Koutsu-Sho-ni-okeru Shingata-Koronauirusu-Kansensho-heno Taiou-joukyou 2020-nen-7-gatsu-3-nichi Jiten." Accessed October 6, 2020. www.mlit.go.jp/common/001351363.pd.

MLIT. "Shingata-Koronauirusu-Kansensho-ni-tomonau Kankei-Gyoukai-no Eikyo-ni-tsuite." www.mlit.go.jp/kikikanri/content/001348188.pdf.

National Institute of Infectious Diseases. "Shingata-Koronauirusu SARS-CoV-2-no Genomu-Bunshi-Ekigaku-Chousa." www.niid.go.jp/niid/images/research_info/genome-2020_SARS-CoV-MolecularEpidemiology.pdf.

NHK. "Machino-hitode-ha? Zenkoku 18-chiten Gurafu." Accessed October 7, 2022. https://www3.nhk.or.jp/news/special/coronavirus/outflow-data/ Accessed.

OECD. "Maskenpflicht in Handel und Öffis fällt ab Juni, Wien geht strengeren Weg." Accessed August 30, 2022. www.oecd.org/cfe/regionaldevelopment/Japan.pd.

ORF. "300 Mio. Euro Mehr Für Öffentlichen Verkehr." May 22, 2020. https://orf.at/stories/3166690/.

PASMO Inc. "PASMO Basu-Jigyousha." Accessed August 30, 2022. www.pasmo.co.jp/area/bus.

RND. "Coronavirus-Krise: Stadt Wien Spendiert Senioren Freie Taxi-Fahrten." March 26, 2020. www.rnd.de/panorama/coronavirus-krise-stadt-wien-spendiert-senioren-freie-taxi-fahrten-J2O4TLZS5YFQEQJVAINOP67XMI.htm.

Shibayama, Takeru. "Competence Distribution and Policy Implementation Efficiency Towards Sustainable Urban Transport: A Comparative Study." *Research in Transportation Economics* 83 (2020). https://doi.org/10.1016/j.retrec.2020.100939.

Springer, Gudrun. "Maskenpflicht in Handel Und Öffis Fällt Ab Juni, Wien Geht Strengeren Weg." *Der Standard*, May 24, 2022. www.derstandard.at/story/2000136002595/maskenpflicht-im-handel-und-oeffis-faellt-ab-juni-impfpflicht-ruh.

Stadt Wien. "Stadtgebiet Nach Nutzungsklassen Und Bezirken 2022." 2022. Accessed October 6, 2022. www.wien.gv.at/statistik/lebensraum/tabellen/nutzungsklassen-bez.htm.

Tokyo Metro Co. Ltd. "News Release." www.tokyometro.jp/news/images_h/metroNews220707_2.pd.

Tokyu Bus Corporation. "Shinya-Kyuko-Basu oyobi Tsukin-Kosoku-Basu Haishi-no Oshirase." 2022. www.tokyubus.co.jp/news/002670.htm.

Vienna City Administration Municipal Dept. 18. *STEP 2025. Thematic Concept: Urban Mobility Plan Vienna*. Werkstattbericht 155.

Vienna Online. "80 Prozent Weniger Fahrgäste: Wiener Linien Passen Fahrplan an." 2020. Accessed October 7, 2022. www.vienna.at/80-prozent-weniger-fahrgaeste-wiener-linien-passen-fahrplan-an/656154.

Vienna Online. "Coronavirus Wiener Linien Passen Fahrplan an." Accessed October 7, 2022. www.vienna.at/coronavirus-wiener-linien-passen-fahrplan-an/655396.

Vienna Online. "Coronavirus: Bis Zu 40 Prozent Weniger Fahrgäste Bei Den Wiener Linien." Accessed October 7, 2022. www.vienna.at/coronavirus-bis-zu-40-prozent-weniger-fahrgaeste-bei-den-wiener-linien/655603.

Vienna Online. "Wiener Linien Vermelden 60 Prozent Weniger Fahrgäste Wegen Coronakrise." 2020. Accessed October 7, 2022. www.vienna.at/wiener-linien-vermelden-60-prozent-weniger-fahrgaeste-wegen-coronakrise/655783.

Vienna Online. "Nacht-U-Bahn Fährt in Wien Wieder." Accessed October 7, 2022. www.vienna.at/nacht-u-bahn-faehrt-in-wien-wieder/703393.

Wiener Linien. "Zahlen & Fakten Betriebsangaben 2019." www.wienerlinien.at/media/files/2020/wl_betriebsangaben_2019_deutsch_358274.pdf.

CHAPTER 4:

Pandemic and Urban Culture

Displaced Youth and Culture: Informal Art and Culture During the COVID-19 Measures in Vienna and Future Potentials for Public Space

Fabian Dembski

Introduction

Austrian government leaders were optimistic and promised "a light at the end of the tunnel" when the first COVID-19 vaccines became available.[1] What nobody knew at the time was that we would be going from one tunnel to another! As the waves of infections subsided and the course of the disease became milder, war broke out in Ukraine almost simultaneously followed by high inflation and skyrocketing gas prices. Times got tougher for the established arts – that is, the institutions of theatres, concert halls, museums, and galleries in Vienna. Anyone who visited a theatre, concert or opera in Vienna in the months following the end of the lockdowns and access restrictions, could see that many seats remained empty. This was not only the case in Vienna and Austria, but also in many other European countries. Audiences were slow to return to the major venues after all the restrictions of the Corona years, and it was not only the media that wondered whether things would ever be the same again.

"Austria as a nation of art and culture" is a concept politicians, companies and tourism organisations like to use when it comes to highlighting the advantages of Austria as a business location or a tourism destination.[2] But it is also a concept with substance that extends from so-called high culture in the federal capital Vienna and the provincial capitals to initiatives in the smallest communities. Even in times of crisis, the cultural nation is often invoked, especially when it comes to support from the state.

---

[1] ORF, "Kanzlerrede: Es gibt Licht am Ende des Tunnels."
[2] Austrian Federal Ministry of Labour and Economy, "Kulturtourismus in Österreich."

So far, the federal government has had to provide an additional 450 million euros (2020 and 2021)[3] for arts and culture in the wake of the COVID-19 crisis. This raises the question not only of how long we can afford to keep supporting the cultural nation, but also of how it can continue to develop and establish in this so-called "new reality".

However, not only art and culture, but also adolescents and young adults suffered particularly from the COVID-19 crisis and related governmental measures. Lockdowns and contact restrictions not only often increased the feeling of loneliness, but mental illness also rose abruptly among the young (Koubek et al., 2022).[4] Prior to the outbreak of the pandemic, schools, universities and other educational institutions, as well as private apartments, clubhouses, cafés, theatres and concert halls were commonly used by young people, but all of a sudden they were no longer accessible. As such, it is not surprising that from the summer of 2020 at the latest, young people began organising themselves and increasingly used public spaces, — especially in the centre of Vienna and in other densely populated areas — in their free time and adapted them for their own purposes.[5] Although this was mostly illegal or semi-legal, it became at least more or less tolerated relatively soon after the strictest lockdown conditions were imposed.

The use of public space by young people peaked in the summer of 2021, but with increasing conflicts that resulted in bans on central locations such as Karlsplatz and The Danube Canal. On the 4th of June of that year 2021, for example, thousands of young people were evicted from Karlsplatz under the pretext of "threatening damage to property and criminal acts".[6,7] This was accompanied by complaints from neighbours about noise pollution, as reported by the media. Even at this point, the idea arose that social problems could not be solved by the police, but rather that new concepts were needed for the use of public space.[8] The Viennese City government expressed understanding for the needs of the young people and in some cases criticised the harsh measures taken by the police, even going so far as to obtain the lifting of certain bans.[9]

---

[3] Austrian Federal Ministry of Arts, Culture, Civil Service and Sport, "Bilanz Neustart Kultur: 20 Millionen Euro an 831 Projekte ausgezahlt."
[4] Koubek, Krönke and Karwautz, "Die aktuelle Situation der kinder- und jugendpsychiatrischen Versorgung in Österreich im niedergelassenen Bereich."
[5] Schrenk, "Wie die Corona-Krise den öffentlichen Raum neu verteilt."
[6] Staudinger, "Partyschreck im Resselpark."
[7] Csisinko and Weis, "Nach Platzverbot am Karlsplatz: Bürgermeister Ludwig will Räume für Jugendliche ermöglichen."
[8] Gaigg and Winkler-Hermaden, "Räumung am Karlsplatz: Eine Party mit Folgen."
[9] Csisinko and Weis, "Nach Platzverbot am Karlsplatz: Bürgermeister Ludwig will Räume für Jugendliche ermöglichen."

At the same time as self-organised meetings in central, prominent squares around the city were going on, similar activities were taking place practically everywhere in Vienna — with an emphasis on more densely populated neighbourhoods and the parks and squares in the vicinity. Common throughout was the practice and consumption of art and culture in an informal, more or less spontaneous setting. Reports documenting these activities are not readily available. There is also little information about the different places that were used during this difficult period.

Consequently, this is the moment to investigate this topic in more detail and to gain insight into the numerous activities of young people. Where did most of the activities take place and what forms of art and culture were practiced or consumed? Which places were perceived as negative and did conflicts arise? In the long-term, which places hold the potential to serve for public and/or informal art and culture? These and other questions are addressed in this study.

Micro-study on the space-related art and cultural behaviour of young people during and after the COVID-19 measures

A total of 54 young people between the ages of 14 and 28 whose life — especially for leisure activities — is centred around Vienna responded to a map-based survey. To reach as heterogeneous a group as possible with varying social and cultural backgrounds, participants were invited to take part in an online survey advertised via social media popular with the target group.

The survey was implemented with the help of the online tool *Maptionnaire*.[10] This is a Public Participation GIS (PPGIS) platform that enables location-based and qualitative data to be collected and analysed from the users surveyed.[11]

59 % of respondents were male, slightly over a third were female (35 %), and the remainder non-binary. The time frame was set from 08/25/2022 to 01/31/2023.

Due to the limited number of respondents, the results can be described more as sample findings than as a representative study. Nevertheless, it seems that initial conclusions can be drawn and trends derived. The difficulty with online surveys such as Maptionnaire, is that the target group in the geographically defined area is not easy to reach. Consequently, it was only with great effort and by using social networks such as Facebook, Instagram or WhatsApp groups as well

---

[10] Maptionnaire, "Maptionnaire — a hassle-free citizen engagement platform."
[11] Brown and Kyttä, "Key issues and research priorities for public participation GIS (PPGIS): A synthesis based on empirical research."

as personal contacts (for example parents or teachers at schools and universities) that we were able to reach 54 respondents.

In this research the focus of the questions was on the use of public space for the practice and/or consumption of art and culture in and around Vienna during the COVID-19 crisis and the corresponding lockdowns and access restrictions. Users were also surveyed about their behaviour after these measures had come to an end in 2022, and about the future potential for public art and culture in urban space.

Survey and structure

The questionnaire could be filled out online, was available in German and English, and consisted of 20 questions. In addition to geo-based data (GIS) and basic information i.e. age, gender, education, and employment status, were questions about the impact of the lockdowns and access restrictions on social life, on artistic activities, on the period of these activities, and on conflicts in public spaces. The question of the commercialisation of art and free access to cultural activities was also addressed.

The geo-referenced responses could be provided online via interactive maps of the city of Vienna and its environs. For example, by selecting a tool respondents were able to define areas to mark their places of activities during and after the COVID-19 measures.

Furthermore, the maps provided on Maptionnaire allowed respondents to zoom in and to search for specific addresses to improve usability. As a first question of this type, the respondents were asked about their leisure time behaviour or the public spaces used for this purpose during the lockdowns.

Additionally, respondents were asked about the public spaces where young people consumed art and culture during this period. Examples deliberately included more established activities (such as music and dance), as well as more youth cultural activities (such as graffiti and performances). Geo-referenced answers regarding a given respondent's own art or cultural activities in public spaces could also be defined.

Cities or their public spaces also harbour risks for conflict or other dangerous situations, particularly for young people. Respondents could provide general information on this in a question with a slider (from never to frequently) and then locate the corresponding areas geographically on the city map in a follow-up question.

The next block of questions addressed user behavior in public places visited by the respondents in 2022 after the Corona restrictions had been lifted. Respondents were also asked about locations that, in their opinion, could provide potential for public art and culture in the future.

Results

The question about the personal impact of the lockdowns on the respondents' social life indicated that it had been significant. The majority (62.5%) considered the impact to have been "very strong", just over 15% "fairly strong" (16.67%) and just under 5% "strong" (4.17%). Slightly less than 10% perceived the measures as "marginal" (8.33%), almost 5% as "moderate" (4.17%) with the remaining 4.17% not being at all affected (Table 1).

"very strong"	62.5%
"fairly strong"	16.67%
"strong"	4.17%
"marginal"	8.33%
"moderate"	4.17%
"not affected at all"	4.17%

Table 1: Personal impact of the lockdowns on the respondents' social life

When asked about their consumption of arts and culture during the lockdowns compared to before the pandemic, again the majority felt "relatively strongly" to "very strongly" constrained (63.64%) with just under a fifth feeling only "a little" to "moderately" constrained (18.18%) and the remainder feeling not at all restrained (18.18%) (Table 2).

"relatively strongly" to "very strongly" constrained	63.64%
"a little" to "moderately" constrained	18.18%
"not affected at all"	18.18%

Table 2: Consumption of arts and culture during the lockdowns compared to before the pandemic

The restrictions and the resulting long-lasting bans on indoor activities led to the respondents shifting their leisure activities to the open spaces of the city. Here, activities were heavily concentrated on public spaces south of The Danube and in green space areas such as the Wienerwald (the Vienna Woods partially within the 14th and 19th districts), the Lainzer Tiergarten (a wildlife preserve in the 13th district) and the Prater (a large park in the 2nd district), but also in parts of the 3rd, 10th and 11th districts, and in less densely built-up areas (for example the Laaer Berg hill, and the Kurpark Oberlaa — a large green space adjoining the Oberlaa health resort — both in the 10th district). In more densely built-up areas, the focus of activities was in the 2nd and 3rd districts adjacent to the northeast of the city centre, and in the 4th, 5th and 10th districts south of the inner city (Figure 1).

The passive consumption of art and culture by the respondents (Figure 2) largely focused on the inner districts of the city. Namely the Praterstern railway station and its surroundings in the 2nd district, Karlsplatz in the 4th district, the Wiental i.e. the area along the banks of The Wienfluss (The Vienna River), Gumpendorferstrasse in the 6th district and the old general hospital in the 9th district (which is now home to an inner courtyard of bars, restaurants and green space) were the main areas of focus. But there were also cultural activities taking place south of the city, namely in Liesing and Erlaa in the 23rd district and Oberlaa in the 10th, as well as in the north of Vienna in the neighbourhood of Stammersdorf and in Gerasdorf in neighbouring Lower Austria.

Just over a fifth of of respondents regularly engaged in artistic activities in public spaces during the pandemic (22,2%), a third were occasionally active and almost half were rarely to not active at all (44,4%). Activities included, for example, performing arts such as dance, theatre and music making, visual arts such as drawing, painting, sketching or graffiti, and poetry and digital arts.

Activities mostly took place between midday and 6:00pm (approximately a third of respondents) and between 6:00pm and 10:00pm (just under a third of respondents). Only a few were active during the mornings between 6:00am and midday (around 15%) or in the evenings later than 10:00pm (again around 15%).

Regarding spatial distribution (Figure 3), participants largely used central locations such as the area adjoining Karlsplatz in the 1st district and the walkways along The Danube Canal where it separates the 1st and the 2nd districts. However, densely populated areas in the 4th, 5th, 6th, 10th and 15th districts were also used frequently, namely the area of The Wienfluss (The Vienna River), the major arterial roads like Wienzeile and along the outer ring road known as The Gürtel.

Respondents also indicated activities in Vienna's periphery. Here, especially in the north-west in the area of the Bisamberg hill and on into the neighbouring state of Lower Austria (in the district of Korneuburg), as well as in the south in the region of the new urban development area known as Rothneusiedl in the 10th district and in the district of Baden, again in the neighbouring state of Lower Austria. In only a few cases (12,5%) did conflicts arise with residents or the police, all of which were related to noise.

Another question looked at the experience or perception of danger in public spaces. Half of the respondents occasionally experienced dangerous situations and around 8% felt strongly affected by them, with just over two fifths stating that dangerous situations in public spaces either never or hardly ever occurred.

The places that were perceived as dangerous or unpleasant by the participants could also be defined and represented in one of the map surveys (Figure 4). Surprisingly, these places were defined very specifically in the map survey: The area surrounding the Praterstern railway station in the 2nd district, Votivpark linking the 1st and 9th districts, Stadtpark between the 1st and adjacent 3rd districts. Further west, these areas were largely in the vicinity of the metro stations Margaretengürtel (5th district), Meidling-Hauptstrasse (12th and 15th districts), Westbahnhof (15th and 7th districts) and Josefstädterstrasse (16 and 8th districts).

The fact that the lockdowns had a strong impact on the majority of the respondents is not surprising as this coincides with studies that have focused particularly on this question.[12] Equally unsurprising is that the restrictions affected the consumption of arts and culture among the majority of respondents. However, the relatively high level of cultural and artistic activity among the young people surveyed during the lockdowns is remarkable. The pandemic-related restrictions, it seems, motivated many to engage in their own artistic and cultural endeavours. Understandably, most of these activities took place at times other than late at night and early in the morning, since curfews and other restrictions were in effect in the city. From February 8 to May 19, 2021, for example, there was a strict curfew in place between the hours of 8:00pm and 6:00am. Also at this time people who were not of the same household were obliged to maintain a distance of two meters from one another when out in public.

---

[12] Koubek, Krönke and Karwautz, "Die aktuelle Situation der kinder- und jugendpsychiatrischen Versorgung in Österreich im niedergelassenen Bereich."

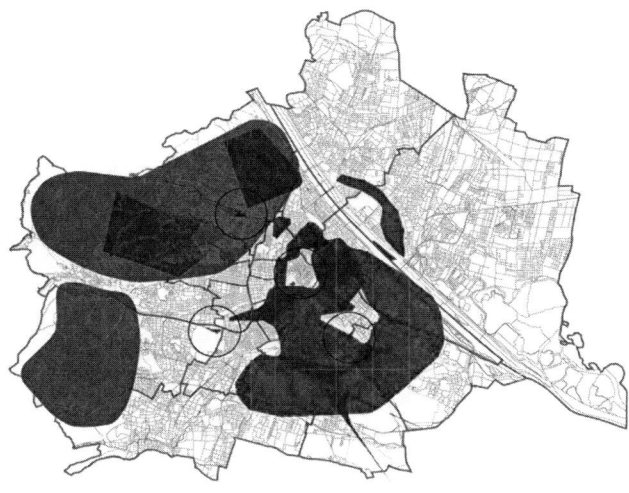

Fig. 1: Spatial distribution of public places visited during leisure time

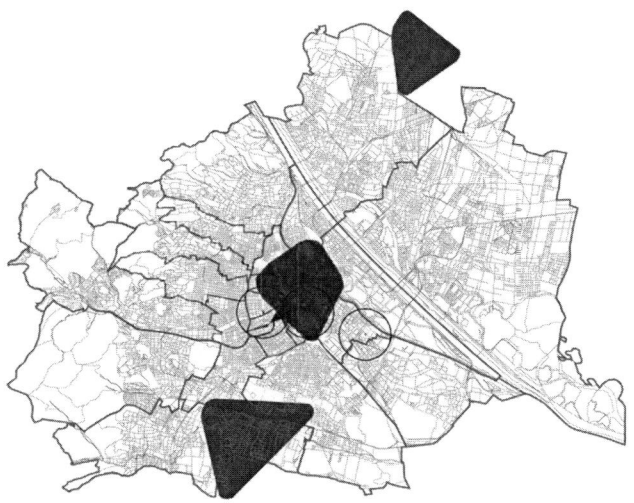

Fig. 2: Spatial distribution of public places visited for passive consumption of art and culture[13]

---

[13] Fig. 1-7: City of Vienna, "Base map of the city of Vienna."

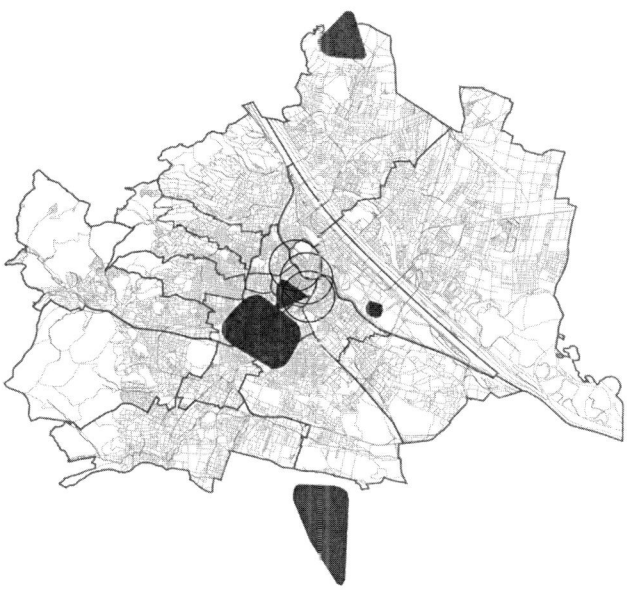

Fig. 3: Spatial distribution of public places visited for active production of art and culture

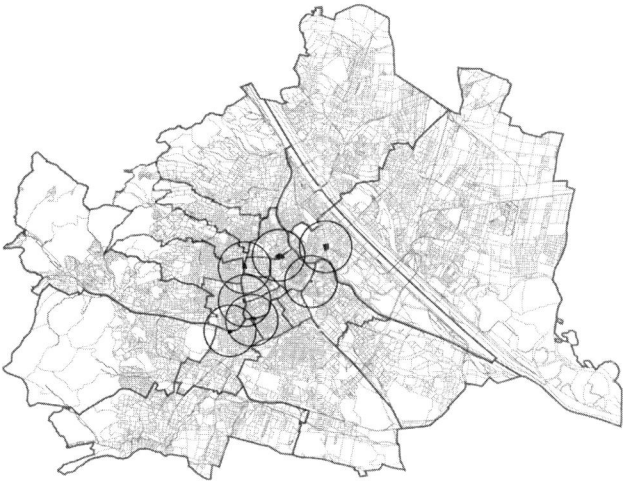

Fig. 4: Spatial distribution of public places perceived as "dangerous" or "uncomfortable"

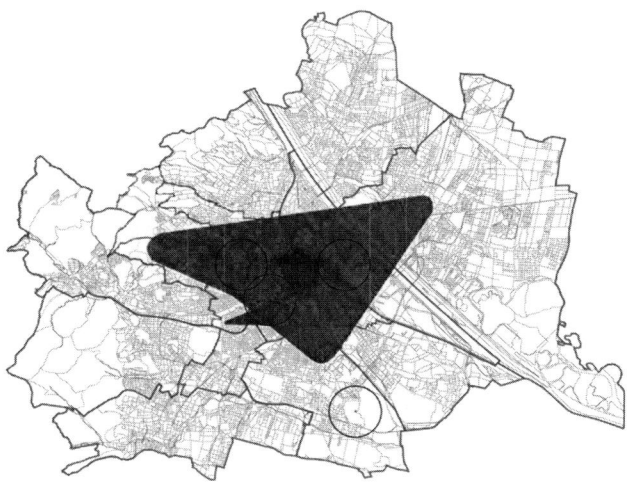

Fig. 5: Spatial distribution of public places visited after the COVID-19 measures

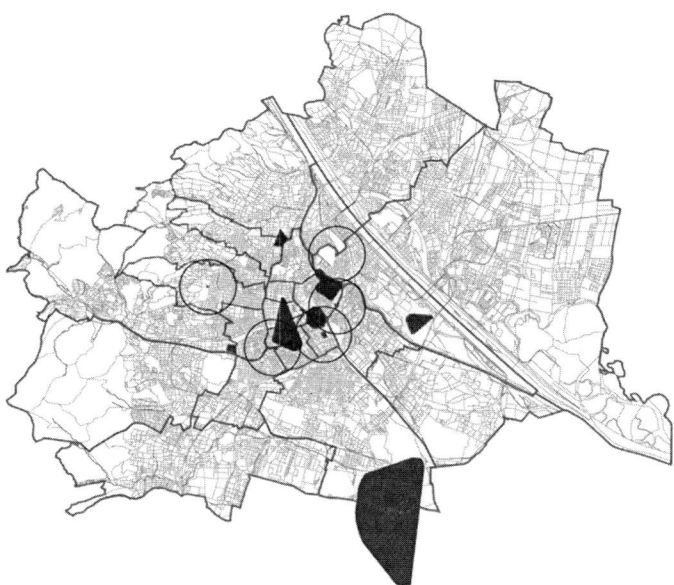

Fig. 6: Spatial distribution of public places with the future potential for public art and culture

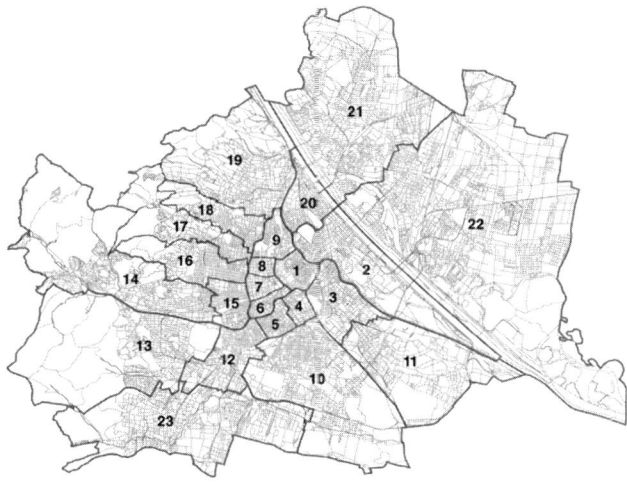

Fig. 7: Overview map of the Viennese districts

Despite these restrictions, the public practice of cultural or artistic activities rarely led to conflicts for the respondents. Reports on this topic have, however, appeared in the media, mostly concerning specific, very central locations, where conflicts are potentially more likely than in the outskirts of Vienna due to high population density.

Respondents were not only asked about their past and present activities. They were also questioned about how they see the future of art and cultural events and how accessible they expect them to be. Two fifths believed that art and culture should be free for all, with no consumerist pressure. The same number want to support artists and cultural workers financially, but believe this should be on a voluntary basis. In contrast, just over 15 % think that art and cultural events in public spaces should be professionally organised and are willing to pay an entrance fee. Less than 5 % think that art and culture do not belong in public spaces. Some arguments were, for example, that art and culture in public space must not compete with other uses, which could, for example, lead to the displacement of consumption-free meeting places in certain places due to these events. It was also argued that there should be more space for young people in public spaces, but that this should be well-organised to prevent decay and neglect. Also the definition of art and culture was questioned and it was pointed out that tensions exist between "impulsivity (sic) and organisation, and between artistic norms and their sublimation". The same respondent also stated that "it would be nice to see less focus on 'street art' – this currently dominates as an idea because it is part of a postmodernist wave".[14]

Public places that are still increasingly visited for art and cultural purposes today are mainly located in the centre of the city (Figure 5, as of 2022). Hotspots here are the 1st district, the adjacent 2nd district neighbourhoods around Taborstrasse and Karmelitermarkt, the Wiental and its surroundings, the main city library between the 7th and the 15 districts along with other areas inside and outside of The Gürtel and in the green space along the banks of The Danube, The Danube Island and The Old Danube. Also to some extent in the 22nd district.

Whereas the locations where young people still spend time today in order to experience art and culture in public space were rather broadly defined, those locations with future potential were more specifically defined (Figure 6) with all of the following featuring heavily: Karlsplatz and Resselpark, which link the 1st and 4th districts, the walkways along each side of The Danube Canal where it separates the 1st and 2nd districts, the western inner districts of the Wiental (parts of the 8th, 7th, 6th and, 5th districts) and parks such as Auer-Welsbach Park in the 15th district, the Prater and the Augarten Park in the 2nd, as well as the area around the Hohe Warte hill near the social housing estate known as Karl-Marx Hof in the 19th. Other smaller parks and squares in more densely populated areas, the area surrounding Oberlaa in the 10th district and south of Vienna, namely the district of Baden in Lower Austria, were also mentioned, this latter being close to the Rothneusiedl urban development area in the 10th.

Summary of results

The COVID-19 era has not passed without leaving its mark on young people. However, the continued heavy use of public space – also for artistic and cultural activities – could be described as a positive effect. Although no detailed data are available in Vienna on the use of these urban spaces before, during and after the pandemic, the results of this survey with its relatively small number of participants reveal tendencies that indicate that public space is being used more today than it was previously. While young people identify locations with future potential for art and cultural activities that were also frequented for this purpose during the lockdowns, they also recognise the need and potential in other places that are not as

---

[14] Responses from the questionnaires (not attributable to specific individuals due to anonymisation).

yet heavily frequented. Furthermore, it is interesting that these also coincide with current urban development areas or are located nearby (e.g. Rothneusiedl).

It is also evident that there is a need for informal and "sub-cultural" places in the city, and — according to the respondents — these should ideally be both free and accessible.

With regard to the dynamically changing activities and uses in public space, more precise and in-depth studies would be useful. However, the survey method or PPGIS is only suitable to a limited extent because representative groups of respondents can only be reached with great effort. Methods and tools such as citizen science, the analysis of mobile phone data or patterns from movement and stationary activities that can be collected and analysed anonymously by cameras[15] through machine learning could provide better and more detailed insights.[16] For Vienna, however, the opportunity exists to expand the use of public space for low-threshold access to art and culture and, in this sense, to create a better and more inclusive "new normal".

Conclusions

One conclusion suggested by observations during and after the lockdowns in urban space and in the post-COVID era, is that public spaces will increasingly be used for art and cultural activities in the future. An evaluation of the survey permits us to identify potential spaces for this purpose. Precise studies or more representative surveys would be required, however, in order to guide and support concrete spatial developments. In the study presented here, young people were surveyed because their activities were the most visible during the COVID-19 measures and were the most publicly discussed. For a comprehensive analysis people of other age groups and from other social backgrounds should also be surveyed on a representative scale.

What is for certain is that free use of public space seems to hold great potential for cities. Instead of feared conflicts and dangers, which were expressed in the media and by some political representatives, positive effects prevailed. This could also support cities in other transformation processes such as the reduction of traffic and the promotion of walkability, as well as encouraging

---

[15] It is legal without recording image data with personal information (such as face or identity), but to analyse the camera data directly using built-in microcomputers and then transmit only general characteristics (such as the type of locomotion - car, pedestrian, skateboarder, wheelchair user, etc.), movement patterns or those of stationary activity.

[16] Zeile et al., "Radfahren und Zufußgehen auf realen und virtuellen Flächen – Das NRVP-Projekt Cape Reviso."

public spaces for cultural uses in a more decentralised manner such as in the sense of the "city of short distances"[17] or "the 15-minute city".[18]

The free use of public spaces, along with the creation of safe areas for their inclusive use appears to be of great importance. The city of Vienna also seems to have recognised these needs and changes in the use of public urban space and is continuing the so-called "awareness teams" for public places that were installed during the pandemic. These teams are supposed to recognise and de-escalate conflicts and thus ensure safe places.[19]

Further building blocks should focus on the definition of public space in the context of spatial analysis for potential artistic and cultural activities, as well as their curation. It is obvious that activities in public space contribute to safety. The livelier a venue, the more likely it is to be used by people who have not done so before and the safer it becomes due to natural surveillance[20]: Many people in the streets means eyes on the streets.[21] This promotes not only free and decentralised access to art and culture in public space, but also walkability in the sense of sustainable cities and livable neighbourhoods.[22] In addition, it has the potential to sustain the so-called established arts by providing new informal access for groups that were previously excluded, difficult to reach or showed little interest.

Bibliography

Austrian Federal Ministry of Arts, Culture, Civil Service and Sport. "Bilanz Neustart Kultur: 20 Millionen Euro an 831 Projekte ausgezahlt." Accessed March 20, 2023. https://www.bmkoes.gv.at/Kunst-und-Kultur/Neuigkeiten/Bilanz-Neustart-Kultur.html.

Austrian Federal Ministry of Labour and Economy. "Kulturtourismus in Österreich." Accessed January 20, 2023. https://www.bmaw.gv.at/Themen/Tourismus/tourismuspolitische-themen/tourismus-kultur/kulturtourismus-oesterreich.html.

---

[17] Beckmann et al., *Leitkonzept - Stadt und Region der kurzen Wege: Gutachten im Kontext der Biodiversitätsstrategie.*

[18] Moreno et al., "Introducing the '15-Minute-City': Sustainability, Resilience and Place Identity in Future Post-Pandemic Cities."

[19] City of Vienna, "Konzepteinreichung für mobile Awareness-Teams."

[20] Hillier, "Metric and Topo-Geometric Properties of Urban Street Networks: Some Convergencies, Divergencies and New Results."

[21] Jacobs, J. (1961) "Violence in the City Streets. How our "Housing Experts" Unwittingly Encourage Crime,"37-43.

[22] Dembski, "Energy Conscious Urban Development. Analytical Design Strategies for the Post-Oil City: The Case Study of Greater Paris," 20.

Beckmann, Klaus J., Jürgen Gies, Jörg Thiemann-Linden, and Thomas Preuß. *Leitkonzept – Stadt Und Region der kurzen Wege.: Gutachten im Kontext der Biodiversitätsstrategie.* Texte 48/2011. Dessau-Roßlau: Umweltbundesamt. http://www.uba.de/uba-info-medien/4151.html.

Brown, Greg, and Kyttä, Marketta. "Key Issues and Research Priorities for Public Participation GIS (PPGIS): A Synthesis Based on Empirical Research." *Applied Geography* 46 (2014): 122–36. https://doi.org/10.1016/j apgeog.2013.11.004.

City of Vienna. "Base Map of the City of Vienna." Modified by Dembski F. https://data.wien.gv.at.

City of Vienna. "Konzepteinreichung für mobile Awareness-Teams." Accessed April 2, 2023. https://www.wien.gv.at/freizeit/bildungjugend/jugend/awareness-teams.html.

Csisinko, Hanno, and Paul Weis. "Nach Platzverbot am Karlsplatz: Bürgermeister Ludwig Will Räume für Jugendliche ermöglichen." *Presse-Service Rathaus Korrespondenz Stadt Wien*, June 8, 2021. Accessed October 14, 2022. https://presse.wien.gv.at/2021/06/08/nach-platzverbot-am-karlsplatz-buergermeister-ludwig-will-raeume-fuer-jugendliche-ermoeglichen.

Dembski, Fabian. "Energy Conscious Urban Development. Analytical Design Strategies for the Post-Oil City: The Case Study of Greater Paris." Dissertation, TU Wien, 2020. https://repositum.tuwien.at/handle/20.500.12708/1452.

Gaigg, Vanessa, and Rosa Winkler-Hermaden. "Räumung am Karlsplatz: eine Party mit Folgen." *Der Standard*, June 7, 2021. Accessed October 14, 2022. https://www.derstandard.at/story/2000127211918/raeumung-am-karlsplatz-eine-party-mit-folgen.

Hillier, Bill, Alasdair Turner, Tao Yang, and Hoon Tae-Park. "Metric and Topo-Geometric Properties of Urban Street Networks: Some Convergences, Divergencies and New Results." *The Journal of Space Syntax* 2, no. 1 (2010): 258–79. https://discovery.ucl.ac.uk/id/eprint/18583/1/18583.pdf.

Jacobs, Jane. "Violence in the City Streets: How Our 'Housing Experts' Unwittingly Encourage Crime." *Harper's Magazine*, September 1961, 37–43. https://harpers.org/archive/1961/09/violence-in-the-city-streets/.

Koubek, Doris, Helmut Krönke, and Andreas Karwautz. "Die aktuelle Situation der kinder- und jugendpsychiatrischen Versorgung in Österreich im niedergelassenen Bereich." *Neuropsychiatrie Klinik, Diagnostik, Therapie und Rehabilitation Organ der Gesellschaft Österreichischer Nervenärzte und Psychiater* 36, no. 4 (2022): 160–64. https://doi.org/10.1007/s40211-022-00437-w.

Maptionnaire. "Maptionnaire — A Hassle-Free Citizen Engagement Platform." Accessed February 12, 2023. https://maptionnaire.com/.

Moreno, Carlos, Zaheer Allam, Didier Chabaud, Catherine Gall, and Florent Pratlong. "Introducing the "15-Minute City": Sustainability, Resilience and Place Identity in Future Post-Pandemic Cities." *Smart Cities* 4, no. 1 (2021): 93–111. https://doi.org/10.3390/smartcities4010006.

ORF. "Kanzlerrede: Es gibt Licht am Ende des Tunnels." Österreichischer Rundfunk, ORF.at. https://orf.at/stories/3179146/.

Schrenk, Julia. "Wie die Corona-Krise den öffentlichen Raum neu Verteilt." *Kurier*, May 28, 2020. Accessed October 14, 2022. https://kurier.at/chronik/oesterreich/wie-die-corona-krise-den-oeffentlichen-raum-neu-verteilt/400912151.

Staudinger, Martin. "Partyschreck im Resselpark." *Falter*, June 7, 2021. Accessed 14. 20. 2022. https://www.falter.at/morgen/20210607/die-polizei-als-partyschreck.

Zeile, Peter, Thomas Obst, Fabian Dembski, Johanna Drescher, Özlem Cinar, and Uwe Wössner. "Radfahren und Zufußgehen auf realen und virtuellen Flächen – Das NRVP-Projekt Cape Reviso." In *REAL CORP 2021 Proceedings/Tagungsband, 7-10 September 2021*, 613–24. Accessed August 15, 2022. https://www.corp.at/archive/CORP2021_147.pdf.

Culture and COVID-19: Tokyo's Classical Music Concert Halls on Their Way Back to Being Monofunctional Spaces

Masayasu Komiya

Introduction

Like other facilities open to the public, the major Tokyo concert halls for classical music had to close their doors during the first phase of the COVID-19 pandemic. Concert halls were considered unsafe because they were spaces not only of music enjoyment, but also of social interaction.

Concert halls for classical music have been a symbol of the modernisation of Japan since the Meiji period (1868–1912). The enormous changes that took place in Japan within this period were due to the transformation from a closed feudal society system to a modern state with tight connections to the world economic system. Japan intended to become a state on an equal footing with European countries, which meant taking a leading position in East Asia. Pushing back Japanese traditions while simultaneously importing European culture were to support this development. European culture was considered the ideal model for the renewal of Japan.

Well into the 1950s, classical concert halls featured mainly the then prevailing Kyoyo Shugi principle, i.e., the formation of personality through the enjoyment of literature, music, and intellectual content with a serious and focused attitude.[1] The decades that followed saw a cautious opening of music halls, not least for economic reasons, and the social component of consuming classical

---

[1] Matsui, "Japanese Literature Tradition of Grasping the Intangible Experience Between Enlightenment and Romantic Legacy: Kato Shuichi's Unique Contribution on Linguistic Sensibility in Society," 4.

music became more important. The COVID-19 pandemic was a major step back in time for concert halls.

This study examines the impact of the pandemic on the concept and function of classical music halls in the Tokyo metropolitan area. We will first highlight the immediate impact of curfews on these institutions, then go on to examine the role and function of concert halls throughout their history, and, finally, describe how the pandemic is about to change these functions.

The study is based on a series of interviews which the author conducted with managers, staff, and connoisseurs of the seven representative classical concert halls in Tokyo,[2] i. e., Tokyo Opera City Concert Hall,[3] New National Theatre Tokyo,[4] Bunkamura Orchard Hall,[5] Suntory Hall,[6] Sumida Triphony Hall,[7] Tokyo Bunka Kaikan,[8] and the Concert Hall of Tokyo Metropolitan Theatre.[9] These halls are all located within the 23 districts (Wards) of Tokyo, mostly in the city centre, specialised on classical music, and venues for large performances with capacities of more than 1600 seats.

The Tokyo Bunka Kaikan and the Concert Hall of the Tokyo Metropolitan Theatre are operated by the Tokyo Metropolitan Government and its extra-corporation. Sumida Triphony Hall is run by Sumida Ward Government, and the New National Theatre by the Government of Japan. Tokyo Opera City Concert Hall, Suntory Hall, and of Bunkamura Orchard Hall are operated by private companies or foundations. This difference in ownership is reflected in

---

[2] Mr. Dr. Dr. h.c. BIBA Otto (Musicologist), Ms. HAMANO Chizuru (Sumida Arts Foundation), Mr. MAEDA Keizo (Chief of Public Relations and Marketing Section, Tokyo Metropolitan Theatre), Mr. SATO Kazuto (Senior Manager, Reception and Ticketing system, Marketing Department, New National Theatre, Tokyo), Suntory Hall Public Relations Department, Tokyo Bunka Kaikan, Tokyu Bunkamura INC.

[3] Tokyo Opera City is the common name of this compound facility, which is equipped with three types of concert halls for classical music (a big one named Concert Hall, a medium-sized and a small one) and an art gallery. Tokyo Opera City is located in Shinjuku ward and is adjacent to New National Theatre

[4] New National Theatre is a compound theatre facility, which is equipped with an opera theatre called Opera Palais , a medium-sized and a small theatre

[5] Bunkamura (Cultural Village) is a compound cultural facility equipped with a concert hall called Orchard Hall, a theatre, a cinema, a museum, shops, and restaurants.

[6] Suntory Hall is a facility with a big and a small concert hall, as its name indicates.

[7] Sumida Triphony Hall features a big and a small concert hall

[8] Regarding Tokyo Bunka Kaikan, see details below.

[9] Tokyo Metropolitan Theatre (in Japanese "Tokyo Geijutsu Gekijo", namely "Tokyo Art Theatre") is a compound cultural facility equipped with a concert hall, a medium-sized theatre, two small theatres, galleries, meeting rooms, and shops. It is run by the Tokyo metropolitan government.

the conception of these facilities and was also decisive for the way they operated during and after the pandemic.

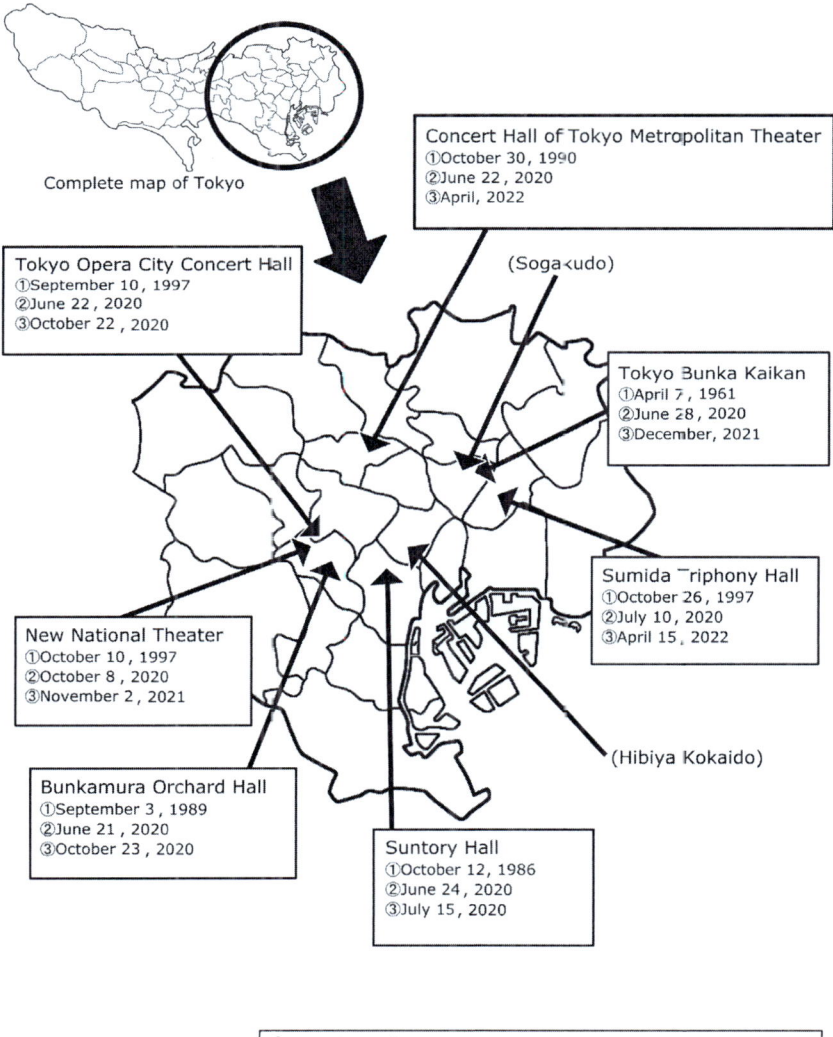

Fig. 1: Classical Concert Halls, Tokyo (Illustration: Masayasu Komiya)

Impact of the pandemic on the operation of concert halls

Closure and reopening of concert halls during the pandemic

Due to the Japanese government's first emergency declaration from April 7 to May 25, 2020 and declarations issued by local governments, most concert halls had to shut down and cancel all performances. After these declarations were lifted, they reopened at different times and resumed their performances in accordance with the guidelines of the governments or theatre associations. Of the seven main classical Tokyo concert halls, all with the exception of the New National Theatre Tokyo halls resumed operation at almost the same time (Table 1).

Bunkamura Orchard Hall (privately run)	June 21, 2020
Tokyo Opera City Concert Hall (privately run)	June 22, 2020
Concert Hall of Tokyo Metropolitan Theatre (run by Tokyo metropolitan government)	June 22, 2020
Suntory Hall (privately run)	June 24, 2020
Tokyo Bunka Kaikan (run by metropolitan government)	June 28, 2020
Sumida Triphony Hall (run by Sumida Ward Government)	July 10, 2020
New National Theatre (run by the Government of Japan)	October 8, 2020

Table 1: Date of resumption of live performances with audience in the COVID-19 pandemic

There are several reasons for the later reopening of the New National Theatre. The first is the nature of its performances. Already during the first wave of the pandemic in 2020, specialists had noted that singing was particularly dangerous because SARS-CoV-2 was spread by droplet transmission. To avoid a higher risk of dispersion, the New National Theatre, an opera house, had to carry out more safety testing than concert halls offering non-vocal concerts.

The second reason is that the New National Theatre is run by the Japanese national government. In Japan, the higher the decision-making level from district or state to the national level, the less flexible its institutions, with privately-run organisations the most responsive. This was particularly important during the pandemic. Thus, the privately run Bunkamura Orchard Hall was the first to open its doors, followed by the Tokyo Opera City Concert Hall and the Concert Hall of the Tokyo Metropolitan Theatre. The publicly led Tokyo Bunka Kaikan and Sumida Triphony Hall resumed operation shortly thereafter. Thus, all privately or locally run concert halls resumed their live concert activity as soon as possible after the declaration of emergency was lifted.

Finally, the timing of reopening also depended on the type of performances planned. It is common for Japanese concert halls, whether public or private, to temporarily rent out their premises to external organisers. Resuming operations at short notice was obviously more difficult when external programs were scheduled. For example, the opening event of the Concert Hall of the Tokyo Metropolitan Theatre was an organ concert produced and marketed by the Metropolitan Theatre itself. At the Tokyo Bunka Kaikan, the situation was somewhat different. Originally, a vocal concert had been planned in a small hall, but this was postponed due to an emergency declaration and ultimately performed in a large hall so that the recommended distance between artists and audience could be ensured.

The situation was similar in the three privately run institutions, Bunkamura Orchard Hall, Tokyo Opera City Concert Hall, and Suntory Hall. The Tokyo Philharmonic Symphony Orchestra, one of Tokyo's most prestigious orchestras,[10] had booked all three halls before. Ties between the orchestra and these concert halls are very close; especially franchise agreements have been signed with Bunkamura Orchard Hall.[11]

Delayed resumption of buffets

Due to tightened conditions, the dates for the resumption of buffets in the concert halls were not identical with the dates of the reopening of the concert halls themselves (Table 2). Not only official authorities but also the audience demanded that special safety precautions be taken, such as a regular air exchange and the possibility of social distancing while socialising at the buffet. To meet these demands, more space and ventilators than usual had to be provided.

---

[10] Some orchestras under a public authority, such as the Tokyo Metropolitan Orchestra (Tokyo metropolitan government), the NHK Symphony Orchestra (NIPPON HOSO KYOKAI: Japan Broadcasting Corporation, a public broadcasting company in Japan), and the Yomiuri Nippon Symphony Orchestra (Yomiuri-Tokyo News company), refrained from concerts with audience until 2021 because they were considered dangerous by these public authorities.

[11] It is a similar situation with the Sumida Triphony Hall. The new start with an audience was a subscription concert with an orchestra, the New Japan Philharmonic Symphony Orchestra, which has a franchise agreement with this hall.

Suntory Hall	July 15, 2020
Tokyo Opera City Concert Hall	October 22, 2020
Bunkamura Orchard Hall	October 23, 2020
New National Theatre	November 2, 2021
Tokyo Bunka Kaikan	December, 2021
Sumida Triphony Hall	April 15, 2022
Concert Hall of the Tokyo Metropolitan Theatre	April, 2022

Table 2: Buffet reopening

The three private organisations, i.e., Suntory Hall, Tokyo Opera City Concert Hall, and Bunkamura Orchard Hall, reopened their buffets more than one year earlier than public halls. Although private institutions also had to comply with regulations imposed by public authorities, they found their own solutions to open earlier and still comply with official government guidelines.[12] For institutions such as Suntory Hall, whose buffet was the first to open after the pandemic, operation of the buffet was as important as the performances themselves as it was part of the corporate concept.

Today's concert halls in Japan are not only important cultural landmarks within the Tokyo metropolitan area, they are also essential social hubs. The institution of the buffet is particularly representative of the social function of these cultural venues. Sociability within high culture in Japan, however, cannot be taken for granted. Cultural consumption and socialising was long an uncommon combination in Japan that did not take hold until the early 1990s, after the bursting of the economic bubble, when institutions became increasingly reliant on new sources of revenue.

To better understand the social function of concert halls in the Tokyo area, we will, in what follows, take a brief look at their historical development, which the COVID-19 pandemic has put to the test once again.

---

[12] Tokyo Bunka Kaikan opens the buffet only with external promoters, not at its own concerts.

Tokyo concert halls: from Kyoyo Shugi to places of social interaction

Emergence of concert halls in the Tokyo area

Tokyo Bunka Kaikan	April 7, 1961
Suntory Hall	October 12, 1986
Bunkamura Orchard Hall	September 3, 1989
Concert Hall of the Tokyo Metropolitan Theatre	October 30, 1990
Tokyo Opera City Concert Hall	September 10, 1997
New National Theatre	October 10, 1997
Sumida Triphony Hall	October 26, 1997

Table 3: Date of official opening of Tokyo concert halls

The first music hall to open in Tokyo was Tokyo Bunka Kaikan in 1961 (Table 3), which means that there was no concert hall exclusively dedicated to classical music in Tokyo until then.

Since the Meiji period, local governments had been promoting the construction of public halls, referred to as *Kokaido*. An emblematic *Kokaido* is Hibiya Kokaido, built by the Tokyo metropolitan government in the central Hibiya part of Tokyo and inaugurated in 1929. Before the advent of Tokyo Bunka Kaikan, Hibiya Kokaido, although originally designed for theatre performances, political meetings, and ceremonies, hosted major classical music performances.

Alongside Hibiya Kokaido, Sogakudo music hall hosted classic music performances. Created in 1890 in Ueno, Sogakudo was the main building of Tokyo Music School (today Tokyo University of the Arts). Being an educational institution, the concerts performed at Sogakudo were part of the college's educational program, but they were also commonly open to the public. Professionals or music agents, however, preferred to perform at the Hibiya Kokaido. It had good acoustics, was attractively located, and could be rented at a reasonable price.

The emphasis on classical music in Japanese culture changed in the 1950s. At that time, Japan began to recover from the shock of losing the war and to rebuild the country. Yokohama, the largest city in Kanagawa Prefecture, was to become the site of the most important postwar cultural institution. Yokohama had been a symbol of Japan's modernisation since the Meiji period; its urban culture was influenced by both Japanese and European elements and was thus considered a particularly suitable location for a building symbolic of postwar reconstruction. In 1954, the local government of Kanagawa inaugurated the Kanagawa Kenritsu Ongakudo, a music hall specifically dedicated to classical music. It was designed by Maekawa Kunio, a disciple of Le Corbusier, with the Royal Festival Hall in London serving as a model.[13]

The inauguration of the Kanagawa Kenritsu Ongakudo was of great importance for other Japanese cultural administrations, especially the Tokyo municipal government. Aiming at the reconstruction of the Tokyo and its return to the international community, it commissioned the construction of a public music centre with a full-fledged concert hall dedicated to classical concerts, opera, and ballet. The new centre was to be located in the Ueno district, which, like Yokohama, was considered a symbol of Japan's cultural modernisation.[14] The design of the music hall was again entrusted to Maekawa Kunio. The new Ueno Music Hall, later called Tokyo Bunka Kaikan, was built next to the new National Museum of Western Art, created by Le Corbusier in 1959. Together, the two modernist cultural buildings created a new architectural landscape in Ueno whose international character was to symbolise Tokyo's new beginning after the war.

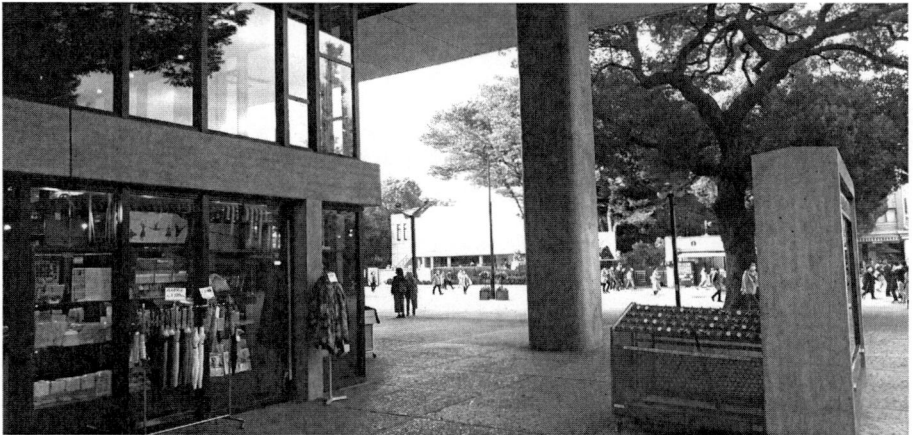

Fig. 2: Tokyo Bunka Kaikan (in the front) and the new National Museum of Western Art (background) (Photo: Masayasu Komiya)

---

[13] Also built in the Modernist style, the Royal Festival Hall was designed as an arts centre and was managed by the London Country Council. Thus, it was an ideal example for Kanagawa Kenritsu Ongakudo for its purpose and governing body.

[14] The first European-style park was established there in 1873, the first modern state museum in 1882, the first modern zoo also in 1882, and the aforementioned Sogakudo opened in 1890 in Ueno.

When Tokyo Bunka Kaikan opened in 1961, it consisted of a large hall for orchestral concerts, opera, and ballet, a small concert hall for chamber music, a music library, meeting rooms, and a restaurant called *Seiyo-ken* (House of Cuisine).[15]

Tokyo Bunka Kaikan concert hall: attempt to create a cultural space a with social function

Architect Maekawa adopted the concept of the Royal Festival Hall also for the Tokyo Bunka Kaikan. This seemed particularly appropriate here, as the aim was to equip the Tokyo building for international music festivals and international congresses. The first floor was to provide a multifunctional space with a large entrance hall, which anyone, including visitors to the park without concert tickets, could enter and which was connected to the foyer of the Main Hall (performance space) located on the same floor. The multifunctional entrance hall was intended to allow a smooth transition between the outdoor space, the park, and the interior space through transparent glass walls. The foyer of the Main Hall, which also was open to the public, was designed as an extension of the entrance hall and the park.[16]

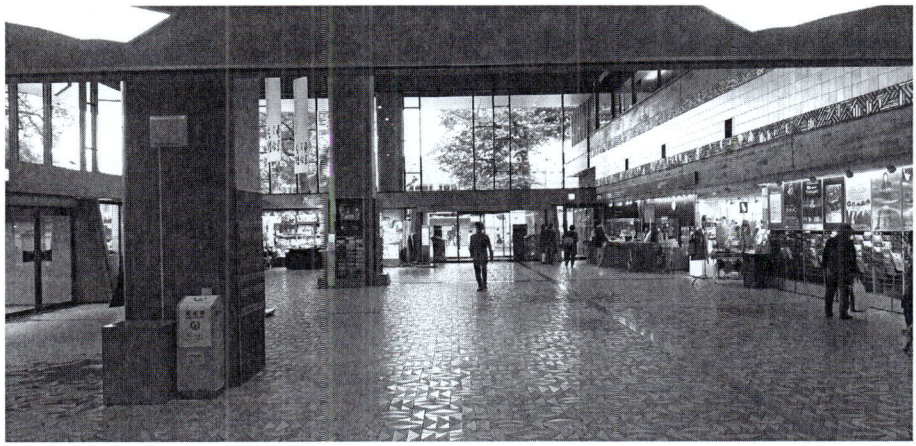

Fig. 3: The multifunctional entrance hall of Tokyo Bunka Kaikan (Photo: Masayasu Komiya)

---

[15] "Ongaku no Dendo wo tsukutta Hitobito," 39–72.
[16] Also in the Royal Festival Hall, the foyer and terrace formed an open public space along the Thames.

However, these new public spaces were not used as originally intended by the architect. The official Tokyo Bunka Kaikan magazine, a platform for famous musicians and music critics, had this to say about the use of these spaces: *"Most concerts in Japan are well organised, but they usually take place in a rather boring atmosphere. (...) In the case of Tokyo Bunka Kaikan, the oversized lobby should be used more effectively. (...) Tokyo Bunka Kaikan should not consider its large hall as a rental space only, but as a space for music lovers."*[17] *"The hall on the ground floor and the fifth floor roof (...) had never been made accessible until the Munich Opera performance the other night. For this performance, the cloakroom and wine bar corners were finally opened to the public. (...) The designers of this hall would have cried"*[18]

In the commemorative journal for the 50th anniversary of Tokyo Bunka Kaikan, *Ongaku no Dendo,* critics complained about the lack of infrastructure and spaces not only within the building but also in its surroundings which would allow social interaction: *"For me as a concert and performance manager, the location of Tokyo Bunka Kaikan is ideal because it is right by the station forecourt and very convenient for visitors. (...) However, I think Tokyo Bunka Kaikan would greatly benefit from stylish coffee houses or restaurants in its vicinity. In Europe,*[19] *there are many spaces where you can enjoy the time after the performance. To enrich the theatre culture, a space where you can enjoy the time after the performance is necessary."*[20]

Yet, for the management of the Tokyo Bunka Kaikan, the music performances were clearly in the foreground, and they paid little attention to the social functions of the institution. Although there was a buffet in the foyer, its selection was limited, and it did not serve alcohol. The restaurant in the complex was run by an external operator and its opening hours did not coincide with the times of the music performances. In addition, concert guests did not step outside the building during intermissions. Ueno Park had been a place for homeless people since World War II and was not considered safe. Also, Ueno was a part of downtown Tokyo characterised by mass rather than high culture, and the immediate vicinity of the Tokyo Bunka Kaikan and the museums of Ueno Park failed to offer a suitable range of gastronomy to a culture-loving audience.

---

[17] Momma, "Hiroi Lobby wo katsuyou shitewa," 310.
[18] Inoue, "Tsuneni Atarahii 'Bunka' kaikan yo!," 642.
[19] In the Musikverein building in Vienna opened in 1873, for example, a restaurant was established in 1914, which played an important role as a meeting place for the public. In 1939, it was replaced by a buffet in an adjoining room of the main hall.
[20] Nakatoh, "Saranaru Bunkaeria e Kitai," 125.

The Kyoyo Shugi principle

However, the lesser importance given to the social function of the concert hall also aligned with the attitude of the Japanese music public. Enjoyment of classical music did not become popular in Japan until the Meiji period and was a completely new phenomenon. To approach this unfamiliar territory, members of the upper class in the late 19th century in particular tried to "learn" this kind of music reception with earnestness and without falling prey to distractions.[21]

This attitude gave rise to a cultural trend called *Kyoyo Shugi* (high educational principle). With the economic boom of the 1960s, *Taishu Kyoyo Shugi* (high educational principle for the masses) emerged. The number of classical music concerts increased, long lines formed in front of the box offices a few days before tickets went on sale, especially for concerts by famous musicians from abroad, and records of classical music sold well.[22] The *Taishu Kyoyo Shugi* boom declined from the mid-1960s and ended in the 1970s with the student movement, which regarded old values such as *Kyoyo Shugi* as superfluous and classical music as old-fashioned or even authoritarian, while rock and pop music, countercultures and subcultures flourished.

Suntory Hall: a new attempt to break away from conventional traditions

A new type of concert hall emerged when private sponsors became players in high culture. The most emblematic is Suntory Hall, which opened in 1986 in Roppongi district, which was redeveloped during the economic growth of the 1980s. The creator and operator of the hall was the famous Japanese beverage company Suntory, whose aim was to gain competitive advantages in the beverage market through cultural sponsorship.

The then president of Suntory, Keizo Saji, was a lover of classical music and a good friend of conductor Herbert von Karajan. Under his influence, Saji had the interior of Suntory Hall designed along the lines of the Berlin Philharmonic Hall. The entire concept of Suntory Hall, created by architect Shōichi Sano, differed from that of previous Japanese halls, especially with regard to the relationship between audience and artists. The arrangement of the audience

---

[21] The attitude of listening to classical music with seriousness originally emerged in the 19th century in German-speaking countries. This tendency influenced Japan, where Germany was seen as the ideal model for a new Japanese empire.

[22] The establishment of the Kanagawa Kenritsu Ongakudo and Tokyo Bunka Kaikan Halls was due to the Taishu Kyoyo Shugi movement.

seats, which surrounded the stage, was a special innovation. In addition, a lavish buffet serving alcohol and a cloakroom were set up in the foyer, along with a souvenir store. These facilities were intended to promote conviviality among the audience, like concert halls in Europe do.

Shōichi Sano developed a seemingly paradoxical concept for the entrance hall, which is smaller than that of Tokyo Bunka Kaikan: *"The design highlight is the main entrance. It is meant to show the two contrasting characters of the hall—the openness of a place that welcomes music lovers on the one hand and the closedness of a special place confined for music lovers on the other."*[23] Special importance was attached to the surroundings of the music hall as a public urban space, with the entrance area of Suntory Hall designed as a wide pedestrian zone.[24]

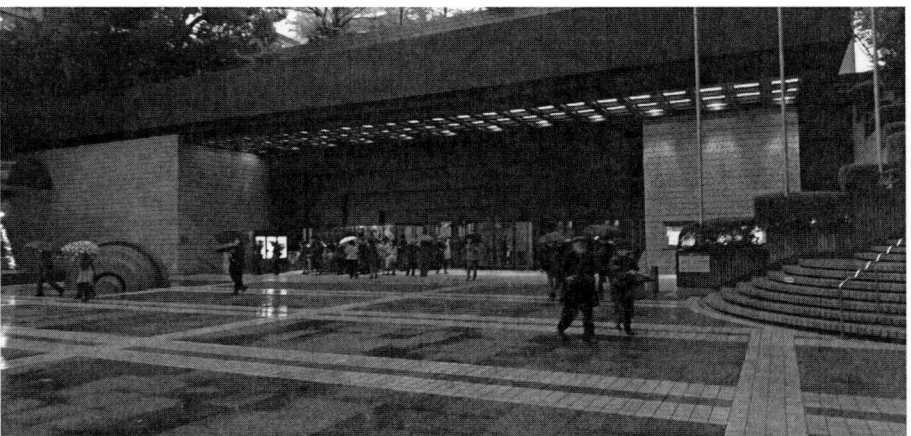

Fig. 4: Pedestrian zone in the front of Suntory Hall (Photo: Masayasu Komiya)

After the opening of the Suntory Hall, the musicologist Hiroshi Watanabe emphasised the advantages of the novel, very European concept: "... entering the hall is through a pedestrian zone designed in a trendy, high-tech, postmodern style (...) during the intermission you drink alcohol (...) When you enter

---

[23] Sano, "Tokyo Hatsu no Concert Senyo Hall, Suntory Hall no Sekkei Shisou," 400.
[24] Although this pedestrian zone is accessible to everyone, on the other hand it is only a semi-public space due to its location (not on the ground floor, but one floor below). Visitors cannot reach the pedestrian zone directly from the street, but first have to go up a flight of stairs.

the Suntory Hall, you have the feeling of being in a concert hall somewhere in Europe (...)."[25]

Moreover, Suntory Hall was equipped with a cloakroom area, which also was a novelty in Japanese concert halls. Taking off coats and depositing umbrellas is the prerequisite for free movement and carefree gathering during the intermission. In the official program booklet of Suntory Hall, a music critic describes the situation as follows. "In European theatres or concert halls, audiences leave coats and umbrellas at the cloakroom, make themselves light, fix their appearance in front of the mirror, and finally enter the interior of the building. This allows them to comfortably enjoy a glass of champagne in the foyer during intermission. In most Japanese halls, however, there are neither cloakrooms nor umbrella stands. (...) In halls that are equipped with cloakrooms, the audience does not use them either and takes their coats directly to their seats. Those who do use the cloakroom pick up their coats before the last act to go home quickly after the performance. In an authentic hall, however, every spectator should take his seat with empty hands."[26]

This comment was written before the opening of Suntory Hall. Following the example of Suntory Hall, all new halls set up cloakroom areas.

Facilities such as buffets, cloakroom areas, or public pedestrian zone outside the building may seemingly have nothing to do with the concert business, but they not only stood for a new kind of concert life, they also intended to help bridge the gap between high and popular culture, and the boundary between private and public space.

Suntory Hall clearly broke with the tradition of *Kyoyo Shugi*, which considered concerts a purely ascetic experience. However, it did not immediately become the space of social interaction that its creators had intended it to be. Since the construction of the large entrance hall and the elegant foyer,[27] large parts of it have been closed and are open only during concerts or special occasions (e. g., exhibitions or open days) due to security reasons.

Following Suntory Hall's model, other private companies or foundations opened concert halls specialising in classical music (Bunkamura Orchard

---

[25] Watanabe, "Chosyu no Tanjo, Postmodern Jidai no Ongakubunka," 163–164.

[26] Kanno, "Sekai no Concert Hall, Europe hen," 493.

[27] Suntory Hall was conceived to break away from the conventional tradition of classical music concert life in Japan, whose symbol was the Tokyo Bunka Kaikan. Finally, the concept of a concert hall with an entrance area open to all people was not adopted in Suntory Hall because the plot was not big enough. Thus, even Suntory Hall failed to break away from the traditional Japanese Kyoyo Shugi principle of a serious, self-contained musical experience.

Hall, Tokyo Opera City). Governments also had public concert halls built according to this new concept (Concert Hall of Tokyo Metropolitan Theatre, Sumida Triphony Hall, New National Theatre). At the same time, Tokyo Bunka Kaikan implemented some structural changes to again increase its appeal to the public. During the renovation in 1999, a modern buffet was installed in the foyer, and a souvenir store was created in the entrance hall.[28] Cloakroom areas were also set up in these concert halls, although it turned out that these were rarely used.[29]

Suntory Hall, Bunkamura Orchard Hall, and Tokyo Metropolitan Theatre opened during the peak of economic growth. The Concert Hall of Tokyo Metropolitan Theatre, Sumida Triphony Hall, and New National Theatre were not completed until the "bubble economy" burst in the early 1990s. During the ensuing economic crisis, investment in the cultural sector was severely cut, and many public institutions, such as the Tokyo Bunka Kaikan, Concert Hall of Tokyo Metropolitan Theatre, New National Theatre, and Sumida Triphony Hall, were forced to self-finance and outsource services. Private halls were also now much more dependent on the services of external music bureaus than before.

One of the survival strategies of the private halls was to rethink their function from a pure classical music venue to a cultural space with a gastronomic offer. The new buffets that were then established everywhere invited people to linger during the intermission and after the concerts. The surrounding outdoor spaces, such as those around the Tokyo Bunka Kaikan, were livelier than before, creating new urban spaces for social interaction.

Even if these efforts did not succeed to the extent that architects and management had envisioned, the concert halls nevertheless did open up to the surrounding space. The economic crisis gave these isolated cultural poles a new direction, modifying them towards becoming more multifunctional. While concert halls did end up becoming social meeting places, they still did not become the pulsating cultural spaces known from Europe.

---

[28] Even after the opening of Bunkamura Orchard Hall or New National Theatre, especially for performances of opera and ballet not a few music companies continued to use Tokyo Bunka Kaikan because of its capacity (TBK: 2303, OCB: 2150, NNT: 1806) and economical rental charges

[29] According to fire safety laws of Japan, visitors of theatres or concert halls do not have to leave their luggage at the cloakroom, although in most cases the fee is free.

The COVID-19 pandemic and the decline in the social function of concert halls

The pandemic put an abrupt end to the tentative social life in the concert halls. Completely closed at first but gradually reopening, the buffets and lounges generally remained closed for much longer. Some 3 years after the pandemic outbreak, some buffets were still not fully operative.

Suntory Hall was able to react most flexibly to the new situation. Due to its tidy cooperation with the beverage manufacturer, it was able to resume buffet operations smoothly. After several test runs, the management found its own solution for this purpose. Not all concert halls were able to follow suit because of their outsourced buffet operation. Moreover, the affected buffet operators themselves were initially reluctant to reopen, fearing low attendance due to the possible risk of infection. Moreover, since the beginning of the pandemic, a large portion of the audience had been bringing their own drinks to concerts.

To counteract contagions and win back the audience, Suntory Hall and later other halls took measures such as regular disinfection of the furniture around the buffet and asking patrons to wear masks. In some cases, the buffet area was bordered by partitions to control the number of users (Suntory Hall), elsewhere, the number of tables was reduced to ensure sufficient spacing, and in some places acrylic panels were placed between the tables. The set-up and positioning of the buffets in the foyer depended, in each case, on the time of resumption of buffet operations. To ensure fresh air, new and powerful fans were installed in many places. In some halls, the consumption of drinks and food was restricted to the outdoor terrace, especially until the official regulations regarding the virus were relaxed. In addition, by government decree, alcohol sale was prohibited.

As a result of the COVID-19-related measures, the buffets and lounges lost the special atmosphere they had all worked so hard to develop over the last 40 years. The flair of the foyers was significantly compromised by the acrylic panels, the new arrangement of furniture, the mask requirement, and the restriction on alcohol sales. Alcohol used to be the best-selling product and, in Suntory Hall, one of the key elements used to advertise great cultural experiences to the public.

While the buffet at Suntory Hall opened as early as July 2020, the buffets at New National Theatre and Tokyo Bunka Kaikan did not open until late 2021, a year and a half after the halls reopened; Sumida Triphony Hall and Tokyo Metropolitan Theatre did not open their buffets until April 2022.

Interestingly, the cloakroom areas reopened even later than the buffets (Table 4), which shows that little importance is attached to this facility. A number of halls, including Suntory Hall, the advocate of the new concert life, have so far kept their cloakrooms closed, first because management wants to avoid crowds, which are considered as an infection risk, and second and more importantly because neither the public nor management had internalised the advantages of cloakrooms described above. The social aspects of the cloakroom area and the advantages of being hands-free in the lounge and during intermissions appear to not have caught on.

Tokyo Opera City Concert Hall	March, 2022
Sumida Triphony Hall	June, 2022
Suntory Hall	------ (except for big baggage)
Bunkamura Orchard Hall	------ (except for big baggage)
Tokyo Bunka Kaikan	------ (except for big baggage)
Concert Hall of the Tokyo Metropolitan Theatre	------ (except for big baggage)
New National Theatre	------ (except for big baggage)

Table 4: Date of resumption of cloakroom activities in the COVID-19 pandemic (Status as of August 2022[30])

Conclusion

In this article, we examined the impact of the COVID-19 pandemic on metropolitan Tokyo's cultural infrastructure, with a focus on the seven major classical concert halls. We have shown that the pandemic turned these cultural centres, which over the last 40 years had tried to become places of conviviality and social interaction, back into monofunctional spaces.

Concerts of classical music did not become a part of Japanese cultural life until the late 19th century. The incorporation of European culture in the Meiji period symbolised the opening of the country after 200 years of isolationism and stood for its claim to a leading position in Asia. The idea of establishing concert halls specialising exclusively in classical music emerged against the backdrop of reconstruction in the 1950s, when Japan ventured into new cultural territory. Unlike European institutions, however, these concert halls were

---

[30] By December 2022, the cloakroom areas of most of the halls were reopened. The cloakrooms of the New National Theatre, however, remained closed. For hygienic reasons, overcrowding by the public was to be avoided.

places of a serious and ascetic engagement with music. The principle of *Kyoyo Shugi* presupposed a focused and intellectual approach to culture and gave no place to social interaction.

Suntory Hall, built in the 1980s, broke new ground. It was no longer just a concert hall. With its magnificent foyer, buffet service, cloakroom, and specially designed outdoor area open to the public, it became a model for a different concert lifestyle. Soon, additional concert halls were created in Tokyo with the aim of turning the musical experience also into a social one. Important aspects were sophisticatedly designed foyers, but also the installation of buffets and the corresponding expansion of the gastronomic offer. Only slowly did the halls develop into places of social interaction.

The economic crisis after the demise of the bubble economy and the dependence on new sources of income gave new impulses to the gastronomies and thus promoted sociability in these places of high culture. Nevertheless, due to the serious and concentrated attitude of the Japanese public, they never became the places of conviviality known from Europe.

The COVID-19 pandemic and the corresponding countermeasures put an abrupt end to any commitment to the social function of concert halls. The hesitant reopening of the buffets and foyers, the accompanying restrictions, but also the acceptance of the measures by the Japanese music public seem to have brought about a renaissance of the principle of *Kyoyo Shugi*. The future will show whether these important cultural centres of Tokyo will remain monofunctional cultural facilities or whether they will be off to a fresh start.

Bibliography

"Ongaku no Dendo wo tsukutta Hitobito." In Ongaku no Dendo, Tokyo Bunka Kaikan Monogatari. Edited by Tokyo Shimbun, 39-72. Tokyo, 2011.

Inoue, Michiyoshi. "Tsuneni Atarahii 'Bunka' kaikan yo!" In Tokyo Bunka Kaikan 30 Shunen Kinenshi. Hukkokuban 1962-1991, Edited by Tokyo Bunka Kaikan, 642. Tokyo, 1991.

Kanno, Hirokazu. "Sekai No Concert Hall, Europe Hen." In Suntory Hall Opening Series Sogo Program, Edited by Suntory Hall, 438-459. Tokyo, 1986.

Matsui, Nobyuki. "Japanese Literature Tradition of Grasping the Intangible Experience Between Enlightenment and Romantic Legacy: Kato Shuichi's Unique Contribution on Linguistic Sensibility in Society." Journal of the Asia-Japan Research Institute of Ritsumeikan University 1 (2019): 1-15.

Momma, Naomi. "Hiroi Lobby Wo Katsuyou Shitewa, Zaidanhojin Tokyo-to Kyouiku Bunka Zaidan, Tokyo Bunka Kaikan." In Zaidanhojin Tokyo-to Kyouiku Bunka Zaidan, Edited by Tokyo Bunka Kaikan, 310.Tokyo, 1991.

Nakatoh, Yasuo. "Hiroi Lobby wo katsuyou shitewa", In Ongaku no Dendo, Tokyo Bunka Kaikan Monogatari. Edited by Tokyo Shimbun, 125. Tokyo, 2011.

Sano, Shoichi. "Tokyo Hatsu No Concert Senyo Hall, Suntory Hall No Sekkei Shisou." In In Suntory Hall Opening Series Sogo Program, Edited by Suntory Hall, 386–404. Tokyo, 1986.

Takemori, Michio."70's -Hoso Chukeisya no Shukuhakunin." In Ongaku no Dendo, Tokyo Bunka Kaikan Monogatari. Edited by Tokyo Shimbun, 89. Tokyo, 2011.

Takeuchi, Hiroshi. Kyoyo Syugi no Botsuraku, Kawariyujku Elitegakusei Bunka, Tokyo: Chuko Shinsyo Tokyo, 2003.

Watanabe, Hiroshi. Chosyu no Tanjo, Postmodern Jidai no Ongakubunka. Tokyo: Shunju Sha, 1989.

Chapter 5:

Urban Green Space and Health Crises

Vienna's Urban Green Space as an Element of Resilience in Times of Epidemics

Meinhard Breiling

Introduction

Vienna's urban green space is the result of an ongoing process of urban development during the last two millennia, mainly characterised by urban growth. Although densifications in core areas in past centuries brought about a loss of urban green, two concentric city enlargements at the beginning and at the end of the 19th century saw a significant increase. However, while this is abundant on the outskirts of Vienna it can be scarce in more central parts of the city. Consequently, not all groups of the Viennese population have the same access to urban green space. Indeed access is co-related to several factors: the availability of urban green in the district, the number of inhabitants sharing it, and individual needs determined by age, gender or income.

The history of urban green in Vienna also relates to the endeavor for public health. A look back shows that green spaces expanded with an improved knowledge of infectious diseases. At the same time, green space was at risk during times of famine and rapid population growth. A lack of urban green can result in air, water and soil pollution, which in turn are sources of many illnesses. The size of a city, the pattern of overbuilt and open space, the communication tools available and the provision of access to green space for urban citizens are additional conditions to how effective urban green can be for the health of its population. Protecting and increasing urban green space, as well as improving access for all population groups, provides better opportunities to respond to local disease outbreaks, regional epidemics, or global pandemics. In March 2020 a new Corona virus appeared in Vienna for the first time and prevailed for three years. It became clear in this situation that green spaces not only provided a source of fresh air, but also helped to maintain the necessary physical distance while additionally serving as a substitute for enclosed spaces.

This article examines the role of urban green space in Vienna as spaces of resilience during epidemic periods. The first section provides an overview of existing urban green space and its distribution within the city boundaries. The second section sheds light on historical epidemics in Vienna and shows the connection between public health efforts and the development of urban green space in past centuries. The third section highlights policies and plans to improve the resilience function of urban green space in health crises.

Vienna's green spaces and their uneven distribution

Vienna has an area of 415 km2, 187 km2 of which is green space[1]. According to the urban planning department (MA 18), the city's green space can be divided into five categories: 1) forests 2) agricultural land 3) meadows 4) parks and gardens and 5) sports fields and campsites (Table 1). Not all categories are present in each district[2]. In the densely built-up inner districts, there are only parks and gardens, while meadows and forests are mainly present on the outskirts of the outer lying districts.

In Vienna, most urban green space is public space. Municipality-owned green space is managed by the *Wiener Stadtgärten* (MA 42, Department of City Gardens, City of Vienna), whereas the former imperial gardens are state-owned and managed by the *Bundesgärten* (Federal Garden Office, Federal Ministry of Agriculture and Forestry, Regions and Water Management). Some large green space areas are privately owned, but subject to local authority regulation. For example, some owners are required to open their green spaces to the public.

Historical genesis of urban green space

The distribution and localisation of Vienna's green space is a result of the historical development of the city (Stadt Wien, 2019). Former imperial gardens such as *Schönbrunn* or *Belvedere* were initially accessible only for the nobility. From the 18th century on they were gradually opened to the public, becoming important urban green spaces. Large urban green areas also include the *Prater* and many green zones on the flood plain west of the Danube, which could not be built on in the past due to regular flooding. After extensive flood-control engineering of the Danube in the 1870s, some of these areas were preserved as green spaces serving

---

[1] Stadt Wien, "Grünflächen nach Nutzungsklassen und Bezirken 2021."
[2] Ibid.

flood retention. Large green spaces such as the *Wienerwald* (Vienna Woods) in the north and west, *Marchfeld* and *Bisamberg* in the north and east and the *Lobau* floodplain in the southeast were only integrated into the administrative area between 1892 and 1905 as "*Wald- und Wiesengürtel*". Urban growth stagnated during the 20th century, which is why to this day these areas are situated on the outskirts of the city (Fig.1). In 1995 it became the "*Wiener Grüngürtel*" (Vienna Green Belt), which is still not finished and work in progress (Breiling and Ruland, 2008). In the 21st century, reoccurring urban growth required a revision of the urban green space guidelines. A "Freiraumnetz" (open space net) aims to connect isolated urban green space to a larger urban environment entity. Thereby, functionality and added quality of urban green is in focus (M. Stadt Wien, Stadtentwicklung und Stadtplanung, 2023).

Quantity and category of green spaces per district

Altogether urban green space makes up 45 % of Vienna's administrative area with an average of 97 m2 per person. This figure is very high compared to other European metropolises[3]. In the first district, the historic core of the city, the share of urban green space is slightly less than 10 % of the urban area. The lowest proportion of green space is found in the districts closest to the city centre, namely the fourth to the ninth, with a share of only 2 % to 10 % of the district area (Table 2). Residents of these districts lack nearby urban greenery and have to travel longer distances to get to green spaces. Inner districts with little greenery are located within the 19th century city area, which is characterised by its dense block perimeter development.

Table 2 gives an overview of urban green space in the 23 districts and shows their uneven distribution within the city. However, these values vary greatly between central districts such as the sixth to the eighth having only 1 m2 of urban green space per capita and outer lying districts such as the thirteenth, which has 492 m2 of green space per capita. In the outer districts there is an average of 119 m2 of urban green space per capita, in the inner districts 20 m2 and in the centre 17 m2.

---

[3] Ichner, "Wien gehört zu den grünsten Metropolen Europas."

1. Forests:

Forested areas occupy the largest portion of Vienna's urban green space (82 km2 or 44 % of the urban green space). They cover the mountainous, pre-alpine Wienerwald (Vienna Woods, altitude 190 m to 542 m). The Wienerwald and the forests of the neighbouring federal state of Lower Austria were combined into a "Biosphere Park" by UNESCO in 2005 and placed under special protection. *(Biosphären Park Wienerwald)*. The forest area also includes the flat alluvial forests near the Danube such as the *Lobau* in the south-eastern part of the city. The latter represents Vienna's 25% share of the *Nationalpark Donau-Auen* established in 1996 according to IUCN criteria.

In addition to the forested areas in Vienna, the city owns and manages forests in the federal states of Lower Austria and Styria, which primarily provide freshwater resources for the Viennese population. Forests are managed by *Klima, Forst- und Landwirtschaftsbetrieb* (MA 49, Climate, Forestry and Agricultural Office of the City of Vienna).

2. Agricultural land:

Vienna's agricultural areas are mainly fields for organic cereal cultivation, but there are also vineyards, allotment gardens and orchards. Agricultural areas cover 57 km2 of the urban area and account for 30% of the urban green space. Vienna boasts 645 farms, one of which is the largest organic farm in Austria. Owned by the City of Vienna it is a pioneer in testing modern agricultural methods. At 30%, the share of organic producers is above the Austrian average of 22.7%. Among the farms are about 100 *Heurigen* farms (family-run wine grower businesses that are legally allowed to sell wine to visitors).

Three quarters of the agricultural land is arable land for grain and oilseed cultivation. Interested citizens can rent plots of 40 to 80 m2 from the municipality at low cost during the growing season to raise their own vegetables in a "self-harvest" project. The main purpose is to promote the pleasure of gardening for everyone while centralising more laborious parts of the field preparation at the municipal management office.

Agricultural land is mainly cultivated by private owners and in some cases as enterprises of MA 49, Climate, Forestry and Agricultural Office of the City of Vienna.

Allotment gardens (Kleingärten) previously "agricultural land" is currently an own category. In the first half of the 20th century, these small gardens were not only intended to provide private healthy open space for the urban population, but also to allow the cultivation of fruit and vegetables and thus alleviate famines that occurred during and especially after the wars . With increasing prosperity, the garden plots (250 to 600 m2) were used primarily for recreational purposes. In 1996, an amendment to the law on allotment gardens (Kleingartengesetz) made it possible to use this type of land for smaller scale permanent housing purposes, indicating the sometimes-fluid boundaries between agricultural land and building land in Vienna. Accordingly, allotment gardens were taken out as a category from urban green space in more recent statistics while they contribute to urban green space in older statistics of Vienna.

3. Meadows:

Meadows stretch over 23 km2 and cover 12% of total urban green space. Originally, they provided roughage for horses, cows and other domestic animals. Horses were the main "engines" for all kinds of traffic in Vienna until the late 19th century and were fed from local sources.

The largest meadows are located close to the Danube and in the outer districts along the forest and meadow belt. The largest single area of meadows is the Danube Island, created as a flood retention area in the course of further flood-control engineering work between 1972 and 1988.

To date, a variety of animal species that had disappeared during the 20th century have found their way back to the city's meadows. For example, 70 sheep are currently helping to keep the grass in the fields closely cropped.

The management of meadows is either done by MA 49, Climate, Forestry and Agricultural Office of the City of Vienna or commissioned out to private businesses.

4. Parks and gardens:

Parks, historical gardens and cemeteries cover 18 km2 and account for 9 % of the urban greenery. The parks and gardens of Vienna were established during different periods. The former imperial gardens and imperial parks such as *Augarten, Belvederegarten, the Hofburg Gardens* and *Schönbrunn* were established before 1800 are now owned by the Republic of Austria and managed by the Federal Garden Office.

Other historical gardens are owned by descendants of noble families (e.g. Liechtenstein, Dietrichstein, Palffy) or wealthy families (e.g. Geymüller) and are only partially open to the public. Many parks of the

first district originate from the construction of the Ringstraße in the 19th century. Most parks in the outer districts of Vienna were created in the 20th century such as Währingerpark on a former cemetery or Donaupark on a former landfill site. New parks, such as Seepark in the new estate Seestadt Aspern, were created to serve current large-scale housing projects.
Most of the parks are maintained and managed by MA 42 *Wiener Stadtgärten* (Department of City Gardens, City of Vienna). These include three Japanese gardens in the 2nd, 10th and 19th districts. Another Japanese garden is located in *Schönbrunn* Palace Park.
The category furthermore includes 46 cemeteries with an area of 500 ha and more than 650,000 graves. They are mostly located in the outer districts of Vienna. The largest one is Central Cemetery (240 ha) with 330,000 graves.

5. Sports fields and campsites:
Sports fields and campsites make up the smallest share of urban green space with 791 ha - 4% of the urban green space. The municipal department *Sport Wien* (MA 51) manages 170 city-owned outdoor sports fields and two campsites. The category includes 21 outdoor swimming facilities, one of which is the historic *Gänsehäufl* (in operation since 1900). At 33 ha, the *Gänsehäufl*, which can accommodate 33,000 people, is Vienna's largest outdoor swimming facility (Fig. 2). It stretches along an old arm of the Danube, which was separated from the main river in the course of the Danube flood-control engineering work in 1875.
Vienna also has numerous playgrounds, three sports stadiums and two ski slopes. Half of all sports fields are rented out to clubs and their members. Furthermore, there is a temporary ice rink *(Eistraum)* in the park in front of the City Hall (in operation during the winter months). Occasionally, ice skating is also possible on the frozen Danube.

Table 1: The five types of urban green space present within the city boundaries of Vienna

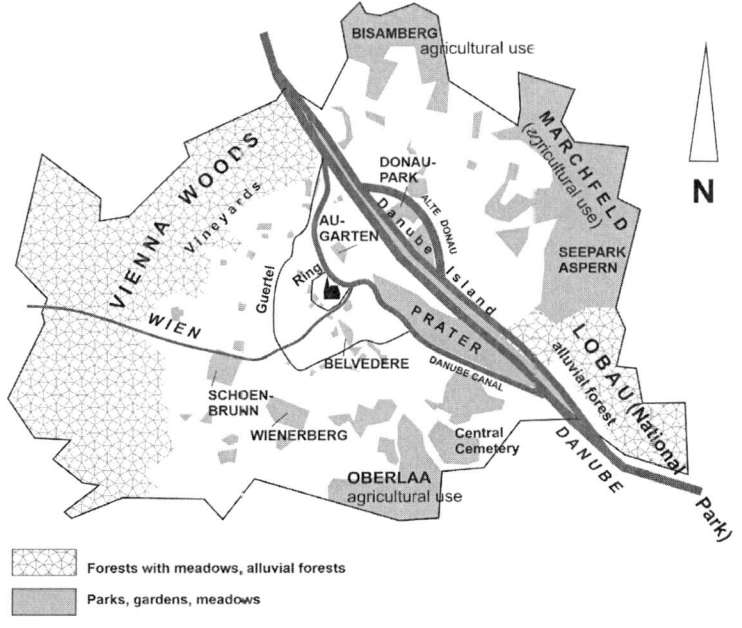

Fig.1: Green spaces in Vienna (Illustration: Meinhard Breiling)

District	Area (ha)	Population 2021	Urban Green 2021	Forests	Agriculture	Meadows	Parks, Gardens	Sports fields, campsites	Urban Green (m2) p. p. 2021
Vienna	41488	1.920.949	18.660	8.159	5.685	2.257	1.770	791	97
1. Innere Stadt (City Centre)	287	15.867	27	-	-	-	27	-	17
2. Leopoldstadt	1924	105.237	675	303	15	66	98	193	64
3. Landstraße	740	93.248	110	4	2	12	80	12	12
4. Wieden	178	33.075	18	-	-	-	12	6	5
5. Margareten	201	54.373	9	-	-		8	0	2
6. Mariahilf	146	31.336	3	-	-	-	3	-	1
7. Neubau	161	31.683	4	-	-	-	4	-	1
8. Josefstadt	109	24.365	2	-	-	-	2	-	1
9. Alsergrund	297	41.812	22	-	-	-	21	1	5
10. Favoriten	3183	210.573	1.440	112	907	119	220	83	68
11. Simmering	2326	105.022	924	102	414	71	307	30	88
12. Meidling	810	96.998	101	2	6	13	73	8	10
13. Hietzing	3772	53.903	2.651	2.073	23	368	169	18	492
14. Penzing	3376	93.366	2.022	1.666	35	211	85	25	217
15. Rudolfsheim-F.	392	76.137	34	-	-	-	23	10	4
16. Ottakring	867	102.480	261	198	10	9	30	15	25
17. Hernals	1139	56.488	602	470	20	59	27	26	107
18. Währing	635	51.327	171	91	4	17	51	9	33
19. Döbling	2494	73.861	1.190	646	355	101	66	23	161
20. Brigittenau	571	85.264	51	2	-	7	31	10	6
21. Floridsdorf	4444	173.916	1.781	261	1.097	216	134	74	102
22. Donaustadt	10230	198.806	5.609	1.690	2.623	866	222	207	282
23. Liesing	3206	111.812	952	538	175	122	78	39	85

Table 2: Distribution and types of urban green space (districts in Vienna) [4]

Table 2 indicates that eight out of 23 districts in Vienna have less than 10 % of the average per capita green or a maximum 6 m2 of urban green available. While five districts with scarce urban green space (4th, 6th, 7th, 8th, 9th) are districts with above average income, three districts (5th, 15th, 20th) are more vulnerable as the average earning of their inhabitants is considerably below the average for Vienna.[5]

The five types of urban green relate to urban planning land use categories and their dominant character as predominantly green space (Stadt Wien, MA18). They constituted 44.98 % of the total area of Vienna in 2021, having been 48.25 % in 2001 including allotment gardens or 45.21 % without. This indicates an average annual transformation of 0.01 % urban space or 5 ha to

---

[4] Stadt Wien, "Grünflächen nach Nutzungsklassen und Bezirken 2021."
[5] Winterer, "Zu wenig Grün für alle."

overbuilt area during the past two decades and very modest change. Changes relate mainly to the conversion from agricultural land either to building land or forest land. Splitting up urban green space into the five categories we find more change. Forests increased by 9 % from 7504 to 8159 ha, parks by 9 % from 1622 to 1770 ha and sport fields by 3 % from 765 to 791 ha. Agricultural land decreased by 13 % from 6506 to 5685 ha and meadows by 2 % from 2358 to 2257 ha.

Previous epidemics and urban green spaces

Urban growth, densification within the given limits and urban extension relate also to previous epidemics and show to what extent the (non-)preservation of urban green spaces are related to public health efforts.

Vienna looks back on a 700-year history of attempts to contain epidemics. Measures known today, such as quarantine, social distancing, masks or lockdowns to protect overcrowded hospitals already appear in history. Health and economic concerns were also at odds with each other in the past. Social differences were also relevant for survival in the past: The poor suffered much more than the wealthy, who could more easily escape to better places such as private gardens or places in the countryside.

Plague (1349 to 1713)

From the 14th century until its end in the early 18th century, the plague threatened the Viennese population about 40 times over more than fifteen generations[6]. The outbreak of 1370 claimed 15,000 lives within two years, which corresponded to an estimated half of Vienna's population at the time[7]. The "Great Plague" of Vienna (1679) claimed 12,000 lives[8], while the population was an estimated 70,000 in 1680.[9]

In 1552, the University of Vienna drew up a first "decree on infection" for the city's officials. A so called "magister sanitatis" (leading health advisor) was introduced to guide the population on measures to contain outbreaks of disease. Houses with sick people had to display a flag with a white cross for 40 days. Only one person per affected house was allowed to leave. Schools and

---

[6] Starting in 1349, major outbreaks occurred in 1359, 1370, 1381, 1521, 1540, 1579, 1633, 1679 and for the last time in 1713. [Velimirovic and Velimirovic, "Plague in Vienna."]
[7] Weigl, "Demographischer Wandel und Modernisierung in Wien, 1700 bis 1999."
[8] Velimirovic and Velimirovic, "Plague in Vienna."
[9] Weigl, "Demographischer Wandel und Modernisierung in Wien, 1700 bis 1999."

markets within the city limits remained closed. From 1555, Vienna demanded "health passports" from distant merchants to prove that they had not visited infected areas[10].

A map of 1684[11] shows that the city, surrounded by a fortification wall, is densely built-up and has hardly any open spaces.

The Enlightenment brought new insights into medicine. In the 1770s Emperor Joseph II founded the General Hospital on a site outside the city walls, which was equipped with extensive open green spaces inside the large courtyards[12]. As part of his hygienic efforts, he also opened up private gardens and haunting grounds such as the *Augarten, Belvedere, Prater* and the parks at *Schönbrunn* to the public.[13]

Cholera (1831 to 1873)

After the end of the plague, epidemics such as smallpox, typhoid and cholera led to high mortalities in 19th century Vienna[14]. Today, Cholera is considered as an epidemic related to impacts of industrialisation and fast urban development in the 19th century such as bad water quality, high building density and the lack of hygiene measures.

Cholera broke out in Vienna in 1831, 1836, 1849, 1854/55, 1866 and 1873 claiming 18,000 lives in total[15]. Quarantine measures could not contain the cholera because the virus did not spread through human contact but through water. Cholera occurred mainly during Danube floods or also in connection with military troop movements. When returning soldiers from the Austro-Prussian War (1866) fell ill with cholera, the *Augarten* (2nd district) was converted into an emergency hospital area.

Increasing knowledge about the spread of cholera led to improved sanitation and urban hygiene. The experience with cholera was a major reason why

---

[10] Velimirovic and Velimirovic, "Plague in Vienna."
[11] Suttinger, "Wienn in Österreich/Auff Ihro Keyserliche Mayest: Allergnädigsten Befehing/ in Grundt Gelegt Und in Gegenwärtigen Riß Verfertiget."
[12] Czech, "Joseph II. und die Erste Wiener Medizinische Schule."
[13] Koszteczky, "Die Geschichte der Wiener Grünflächen im Zusammenhang mit dem sozialen Wandel ihrer BenützerInnen," 44.
[14] Weigl, "Epidemien Statistik – Lieferung 8, Historischer Atlas der Stadt Wien."
[15] "Origins of the current seventh cholera pandemic."

the first high-spring pipeline to supply Vienna with fresh water from the Alps was built in October 1873[16], followed by a second high-spring pipeline in 1910.

Tuberculosis (1787 to 1950)

Like cholera, tuberculosis is linked to rapid urbanisation in the second half of the 19th century. The disease was caused, among other things, by poor urban living conditions (high building densities), poor nutrition, a lack of sunlight thus vitamin deficiency (especially vitamin D), and polluted air[17]. For this reason, it was mainly the working class and among them numerous immigrants who were affected. Mortality was more than twice as high in the densely populated working-class districts than in the wealthy first district: In 1904 for example, Favoriten (10th) recorded 26.44 deaths followed by Ottakring (16th) with 21.11 deaths and Innere Stadt (1st district) with 9.35 deaths per 1000 inhabitants[18].

Better housing conditions, vaccines and other treatments, the establishment of pulmonological departments in hospitals or special sanatoria such as *Baumgartner Höhe* (1910) with its spacious green areas, but also the extension of urban green spaces contributed to the decline of tuberculosis in the first decades of the 20th century.

The preservation of *Wienerwald* (Vienna Woods) from deforestation took a special role in this. The imperial administration responsible for the *Wienerwald* initially intended to fill the empty state budgets by clear-cutting large areas of the forest. An environmental movement led by the journalist Josef Schöffel and supported by the City of Vienna and municipalities of the surrounding Lower Austria, succeeded in 1872 in transferring the management of the forest to public authorities and thus to save them as an extensive public green space[19].

The establishment of the *Wald- und Wiesengürtel* (forest and meadows belt) by the City of Vienna in 1905 including the *Wienerwald* was decisive for the current structure of urban green and its high share of agriculture and forestry[20].

---

[16] The last outbreak of cholera coincided with the 5th World's Fair in Vienna in 1873. The planned fresh water supply had been set up a year too late. Instead of the expected 20 million visitors, only seven million guests came (Seydel, "Visions & New Beginnings – 150 Years of the Vienna World's Fair.").

[17] Dietrich-Daum, *Die "Wiener Krankheit": Eine Sozialgeschichte der Tuberkulose in Österreich.*

[18] Teleky, "Die Sterblichkeit an Tuberkulose in Österreich 1873–1904."

[19] Koszteczky, "Die Geschichte der Wiener Grünflächen im Zusammenhang mit dem sozialen Wandel ihrer BenützerInnen."

[20] Breiling and Ruland, "The Vienna Green Belt: From Localised Protection to a Regional Concept." In Urban Green Belts in the Twenty-First Century.

Against the background of poor nutritional standards and widespread diseases, in particular in poor working-class families, numerous allotment garden areas (*Kleingärten*) were furthermore established by newly founded associations at the beginning of the 20th century. The idea of the allotment garden as a recreational and health space is due to the German physician Moritz Schreber, who advocated small-scale private gardens as part of his health concept for children already in the 19th century.

Key measures to combat tuberculosis were further taken by the Social Democratic city government (Red Vienna) between 1919 and 1934. In addition to the foundation of public health care institutions, extensive green spaces and children's playgrounds were created in connection with 382 newly built large-scale housing units[21].

Influenza (1889 to 1945)

Influenza was an infectious disease that claimed many lives in the 20th century. The outbreak of 1919/20, the so-called "Spanish flu", came to Vienna partly as a result of troop movements during the First World War. The global death toll is estimated at 17 million[22] and 2.64 million in Europe[23]. The estimated death toll in Vienna of 4,500 may be too low, as many Spanish flu carriers also carried tuberculosis and thus widely counted as tuberculosis deaths[24]. In Vienna, the Spanish flu again occurred together with stress factors such as high population densities due to massive refugee flows during and after the First World War, hunger and malnutrition.

The use of parks as urban vegetable gardens, the cutting down of trees in parks for firewood further limited the use of green spaces as recreational areas. In the after-war periods, the use of public green space for recreational purposes was negligible, green spaces mainly served as valuable but insufficient local food and resource supply[25].

After the Second World War, new large-scale green spaces were created in the interest of recreation and public health. In accordance with modernist urban planning principles, these were located in the urban expansion areas

---

[21] Weihsmann, *Das rote Wien: Sozialdemokratische Architektur und Kommunalpolitik 1919-1934*, 110.
[22] Spreeuwenberg, Kroneman and Paget, "Reassessing the Global Mortality Burden of the 1918 Influenza Pandemic."
[23] Ansart et al., "Mortality Burden of the 1918–1919 Influenza Pandemic in Europe."
[24] Dietrich-Daum, *Die „Wiener Krankheit": Eine Sozialgeschichte der Tuberkulose in Österreich*.
[25] Haider, *Wien 1918: Agonie Der Kaiserstadt*.

outside the 19th century city: the *Donaupark* (Danube Park) was established in 1964 on a landfill site, the *Donauinsel* (Danube Island) was built in 1972 as part of a flood protection area, and the *Kurpark Oberlaa* replaced a brownfield site of the *Wienerberger* brickworks in 1974. The banks of the Danube Canal were redesigned as a recreational area from 1988 onwards[26].

Green space policies and the COVID-19 challenge

During the first lockdown in March 2020[27], most important parts of Vienna's urban green space, namely the state-run former imperial gardens became restricted zones. The two authorities responsible, the City of Vienna and the Federal Ministry of Agriculture and Forestry[28], initially held different positions on whether or not to keep Vienna's public parks and gardens open. The former advocated open access, the latter opposed it, arguing the risk of infection. A few weeks after the start of the pandemic however, leading experts classified urban green space as critical infrastructure[29]. Accordingly, all public urban green space in Vienna was managed as such during subsequent lockdowns and made accessible to the inhabitants.

45 % of Vienna's urban area consists of urban green space, which is a high proportion. However, in the context of the COVID-19 crisis, shortcomings such as the uneven distribution of green space in the city became apparent. In times of limited mobility, as was the case during the curfews, the presence of green space nearby is particularly important. The distribution of urban green space, the ratio of sealed land to green space, the type of urban green space, the access provided to urban residents, and effective green space management are all factors relevant to public health. Providing adequate green space for all urban residents is one of the means to better respond to local disease outbreaks, regional epidemics or global events such as the recent COVID-19 pandemic. With the outbreak of the pandemic, urban green space became a temporary substitute for closed facilities such as restaurants, coffee houses, concert halls

---

[26] Koszteczky, "Die Geschichte der Wiener Grünflächen im Zusammenhang mit dem sozialen Wandel ihrer BenützerInnen."
[27] Starting on March 16th, 2020, Vienna and Austria experienced the first of four lockdowns that lasted until May 1st, 2020. The second lockdown was from November 17th to December 6th, 2020, the third lockdown from December 26th, 2020, to February 1st, 2021 and the fourth and probably last lockdown started on November 22nd and lasted until December 11th, 2021.
[28] Full name: Federal Ministry of Agriculture and Forestry, Regions and Water Management
[29] Gugerell and Netsch, "Reflection on the Austrian Newspaper Coverage of the Role and Relevance of Urban Open-and Green-Spaces in Vienna During the First COVID-19 Lockdown in 2020."

and sports centres; at the same time, the health benefits of urban green space became all the more evident.

Urban green space justice

Against the backdrop of the pandemic, the concept of "green space justice" has come to the fore as a necessary principle of planning in many metropolises around the world.[30] The idea, first formulated in the ERC-funded research project "Policy and Planning Tools for Urban Green Justice"[31], addresses the challenge of improving accessibility to urban green space for all city residents, regardless of socio-economic background. The uneven distribution of green space in cities was already a problem before the pandemic but became even more noticeable during the repeated lockdowns when the population's radius of action was restricted to the local area.

The City of Vienna is not only aware of the importance of green space in times of crisis but also of its unequal distribution across the urban space. Interestingly, the key phrase "green space justice" had already made its way into development strategies by 2015.[32]

The STEP 2025 and its guidelines for developing urban green space

The provision of urban green and open space and how to conserve it are some of the most important tasks of the Department for Urban Development and Urban Planning (MA 18) of the City of Vienna. The urban development plan, STEP 2025[33] is currently under revision to STEP 2035 and should be finalised in 2024[34]. The thematic concept "green and open spaces" proposes that every citizen should be able to reach a smaller green space area within 250 m of their place of residence or a larger green area within 1 km. An improved green infrastructure performance is targeted for 12 categories of urban open spaces with linear and shaped

---

[30] Häberlin et al., "Corona: Die Rolle der Stadtplanung für die Krisenbewältigung am Beispiel Wien."
[31] Oscilowicz, "Policy and Planning Toolkit for Urban Green Justice."
[32] Stadt Wien, 2015 Another change in green space availability related to tourism. Before the COVID-19 crisis, some 7.93 million tourists arrived in Vienna and contributed to almost 18 million guest nights with more than 80% share from abroad. Their number drastically decreased to less than one third with slightly over 2 million guest arrivals and 4.6 and 5 million guest nights in 2020 and 2021. This caused particular problems for dependent economic sectors, but provided temporarily more space for those residents living close to touristic sights like heritage gardens. (Stadt Wien, Stadtentwicklung und Stadtplanung, "Green and Open Spaces – Thematic Concept.")
[33] Stadt Wien, MA 18, "Urban Development Plan Vienna STEP 2025."
[34] Stadt Wien, "Stadtentwicklungsplan STEP 2035 – Urban Development Plan 2035."

structures.³⁵ One of the main targets is to become climate resilient by 2040 and avoid the related urban heat island effect.³⁶

As a partial solution, the concept proposes measures such as façade greening, green inner courtyards and roof greening³⁷. The document also points out that areas in municipal ownership such as public baths, open spaces belonging to schools and sports facilities represent an untapped potential for green space use during pandemics. In the sense of resource conservation and "green space equity", these areas should increasingly be made available to different user groups. Although such plans were not sufficiently mature during the COVID-19 period, provisions to counter a future pandemic can be expected in the new version of STEP 2035.

Furthermore, urban agriculture is to be promoted, not only in existing agricultural zones and allotment gardens, but also on small, unused residual areas.³⁸ The completion of the green belt and the interconnection of green spaces are further objectives. The corridors of a continuous green space network are easily accessible green zones, in addition to that, the fauna and flora of the network itself have a positive effect on the urban climate.

The importance of the strategic objectives set out in this document five years before the pandemic was not rendered obsolete by the latter but, on the contrary, strengthened. During the crisis, however, it became clear that the measures mentioned in the document need to be implemented more quickly and that existing green spaces and those to be planned in the future must be adapted to the circumstances caused by possible health crises. For example, footpaths should be widened to avoid dense gatherings of people and more trees should be planted to provide shade for a greater number of green space users.³⁹

Members of the Vienna City Planning Department presented a conference paper (Real Corp, September 2020) in which they stated that the experience from the COVID-19 crisis has encouraged the City of Vienna to pursue the objective of a "robust urban system", formulated long before the outbreak of the pandemic. At the same time, the system should become more flexible to

---

[35] Stadt Wien, Stadtentwicklung und Stadtplanung, "Green and Open Spaces – Thematic Concept."
[36] Winterer, "In der Hitze der Stadt."
[37] Stadt Wien, Stadtentwicklung und Stadtplanung, "Green and Open Spaces – Thematic Concept," 18.
[38] Ibid., 19.
[39] Häberlin et al., "Corona: Die Rolle der Stadtplanung für die Krisenbewältigung am Beispiel Wien," 1275.

allow for short-term measures in times of crises. For example, in the densest districts of Vienna, public space usually used by individual motorised traffic should at least temporarily serve as additional open space.[40] Experiences from these measures should then be incorporated into long-term strategies.[41]

Urban green space as an element of resilience during crisis

During the pandemic, the Viennese were allowed to go outdoors at any time of day "for the purpose of mental and physical recreation"[42]. While shops, restaurants, schools and offices were closed for weeks or months, green space often took over the functions of urban spaces that were inaccessible at the time. In centrally located areas, the number of visitors rose sharply. Some inner-city green spaces such as the banks of the Danube Canal, *Resselpark*, *Schwedenplatz* or *Maria-Theresien-Platz* were so crowded that local authorities ordered the wearing of FFP2 masks there at times[43].

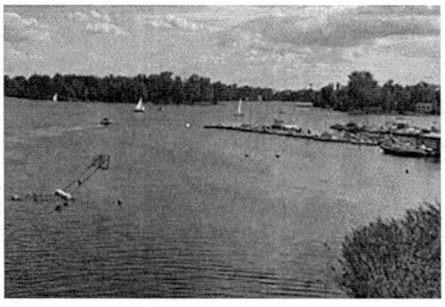 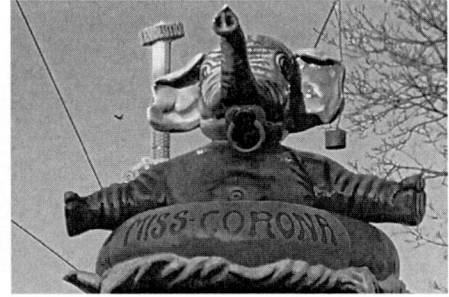

Fig. 2: The Alte Donau Water landscape, view of the Gänsehäufl public baths (Photo: Meinhard Breiling)

Fig. 3: An elephant in the Prater amusement park. In official Austrian crisis communication, the length of a "baby elephant" also served as a yardstick for the 2-metre distance required between two people. (Photo: Meinhard Breiling)

---

[40] Ibid.
[41] Ibid., 1279.
[42] Schmidbaur, "Zweiter Lockdown – Diese Corona-Regeln gelten jetzt in Österreich."
[43] Madner, "Was zu Ostern (nicht) erlaubt ist."

The population's perception of green space and municipal green space strategies

A research team from Vienna conducted a study on the perception of the use of green spaces by the population as a result of the COVID-19 pandemic[44]. The team surveyed people of different age groups living in Vienna and its close surroundings about their personal use of green space and the value they placed on green space after the start of the pandemic. Among the 1012 respondents, 69 % said that having green space close to their home became more important to them, 68 % reported spending more time in nature in general and 67 % reported spending more time in extensive green spaces. 80 % stated that green spaces were important for their emotional health, their mental health and their physical health.[45] The results of a subsequent qualitative analysis suggest not only a shift in preferences within the different categories of urban green space, but also a change in the pattern of usage of urban green space. Green spaces were now considered more significant, and they were used by significantly more people during the pandemic than during pre-pandemic periods. Some consequences of this included an increase in littering and vandalism, and well-worn paths through meadows. The latter were due to the large number of visitors, and to the fact that people sought to keep an adequate distance between each other because of the risk of infection[46].

Public and private contributions to alter the resilience of the urban population

The different aspects associated with the pandemic show that it must be viewed holistically and that strategies for resilience must also be multidimensional[47]. Ecological and social issues have to receive integrated attention. Building on the theory of Charles Rosenberg, an American scholar in science history, Swedish epidemiologist Martin Holmberg considers resilience at three different levels: The first level determines the extent to which an individual can make decisions to counteract personal risk. The second level concerns the social group that establishes internal procedures to minimise the spread of the virus (schools, companies). The third level refers to the municipal and state infrastructure, which includes

---

[44] Tansil et al., "Experience Them, Love Them, Protect Them-Has the COVID-19 Pandemic Changed People's Perception of Urban and Suburban Green Spaces and Their Conservation Targets?"
[45] Ibid., 1004.
[46] Ibid., 1010.
[47] Rosenberg, *Explaining Epidemics and Other Studies in the History of Medicine*.

public health infrastructure and urban green space[48]. Within this hierarchy, the benefits of urban green space in the context of combating infectious diseases can be summarised as follows:

1. Individual level:

- In the context of contagion, outdoor spaces are often safer than indoor spaces shared with others. - Frequent exposure to urban green space reduces stress, improves mood and contributes to better health. - Fresh air in urban forests is particularly beneficial in the case of lung diseases such as COVID-19. - Many people suffered from weight gain during the COVID-19 pandemic with working from home and distance learning contributing to this[49]. Increased weight contributes to an increased risk of infection. Regular exercise outside can help to reduce weight. - Exercise outdoors can compensate for the increased time in front of the screen. - Urban greenery provides a place of escape when tensions between family members escalate.

2. Social group level:

- When indoor meetings are not possible, green space offers the opportunity to meet people (whether for work or for leisure) - even during times of a higher risk of infection.

3. Society level:

- Abundant public green space in the city helps to improve air exchange and to cool the city[50], it provides space for outdoor recreation, and thus contributes to improving public health. (Public provision of allotment gardens or the promotion of guerrilla gardening can compensate for the lack of private green space.) Local authorities that allocate more public funds to the protection and expansion of urban green space generally make their populations more resilient to health crises. In view of future health crises, urban planning must examine the extent to which further greening of areas in existing urban space is possible.

---

[48] Holmberg, *Pandemier Och Epidemier - Från Kolera till Covid-19 I Ett Tvärvetenskapligt Perspektiv.*
[49] Chang et al., "Weight Gain Associated with COVID-19 Lockdown in Children and Adolescents: A Systematic Review and Meta-Analysis."
[50] Pataki et al., "Coupling Biogeochemical Cycles in Urban Environments: Ecosystem Services, Green Solutions, and Misconceptions."

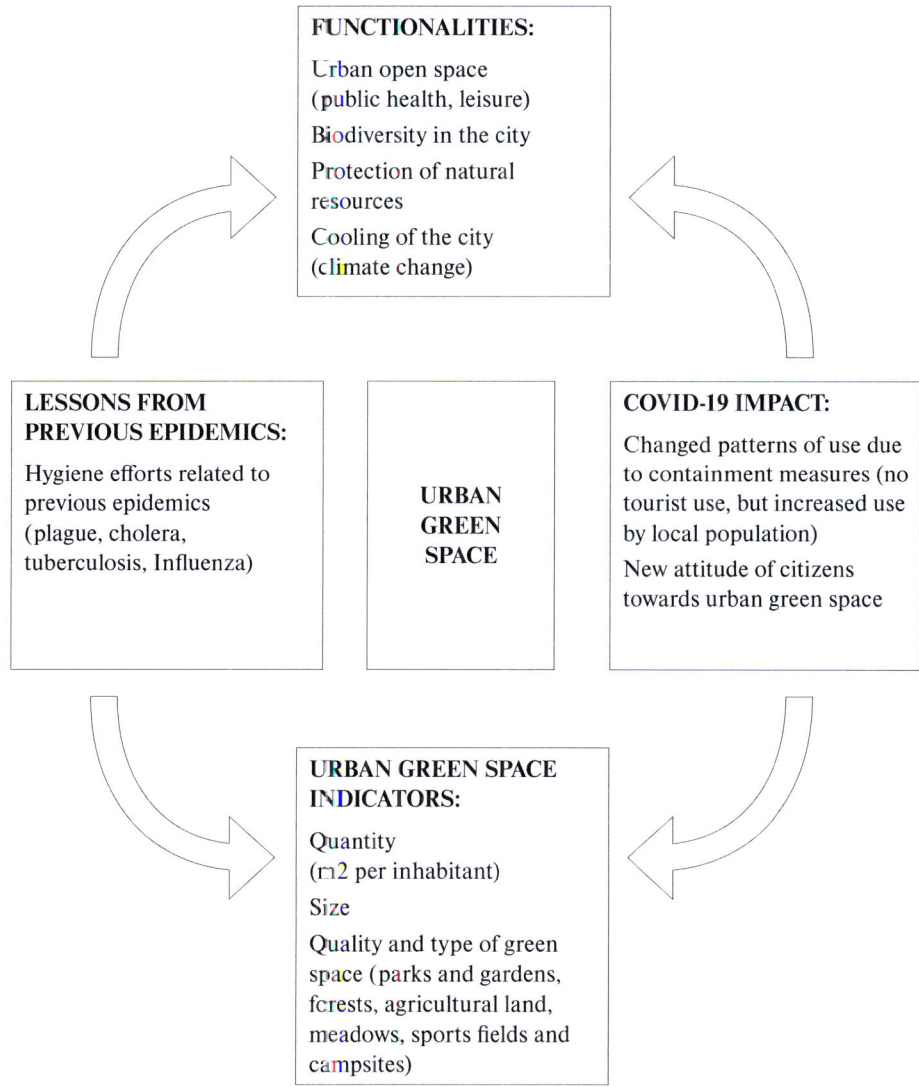

Fig. 4: Functions of urban green infrastructure (Illustration: Meinhard Breiling)

Figure 5 shows the functions of urban green infrastructure which have emerged, among other things, from past epidemics and hygiene efforts in history. The functions of green space have changed slightly due to the pandemic. The quantity and quality of green space is also shaped by historical health crises and may change in the wake of the recent COVID pandemic.

While there is evidence of the benefits in urban green to counter pandemics in a city like Vienna, broadly speaking there is a lack of quantitative studies that show to what extent different categories of urban green are beneficial for risk groups and how to implement measures in disfavored districts. This may result in targeted localised contingency plans for future emergencies.

Conclusion

The development of green space in Vienna is and has been closely linked to public health efforts. Since the 18th century, imperial gardens were gradually opened to a public with better knowledge of hygiene. Findings from past epidemics such as cholera or tuberculosis have contributed to the further development and protection of existing green space.

The COVID-19 crisis has not only shown the importance of urban green space in times of curfews. It has also shown the importance of an even distribution of said green space across the entire urban area. Almost half of the urban area of Vienna consists of green space, yet this is mainly located on the edges of the city. A lack of nearby green space becomes a problem, when the radius of movement of residents is restricted due to legal directives. Consequently, in times of pandemics, access to urban greenery is particularly important as it takes on new functions. During the COVID-19 pandemic, Vienna's green space was not only used for relaxation and sporting activities, it also served to promote health and mental well-being. As gathering places, green spaces were also a substitute for inaccessible closed spaces. Studies have shown that the COVID crisis has changed not only the use of green space but also its perception by residents. The Viennese care more about the time they spend in nature and their access to it than before the pandemic and have an increased awareness of green space close to home.

The developments of the last three years with COVID-19 suggest that crises like the recent pandemic are probably not isolated events, but rather indicators of increasingly unpredictable framework conditions, likely to be aggravated in combination with more frequent climatic or economic disturbances. As such urban green space in Vienna has an extremely important role in consolidating adequate urban resilience.

The City of Vienna is aware of the importance of protecting and expanding green space. The strategy pursued in the 2015 urban development plans goes in the right direction, but the interconnection of existing green spaces and the completion of the green belt must be accelerated in view of future health crises.

In this context, Vienna's urban planning is focusing on creating long-term robustness for the city system, while at the same time allowing for necessary short-term measures.

Bibliography

Ansart, Séverine, Camille Pelat, Pierre-Yves Boelle, Fabrice Carrat, Antoine Flahault, and Alain-Jacques Valleron. "Mortality Burden of the 1918–1919 Influenza Pandemic in Europe." Influenza and other respiratory viruses 3, no. 3 (2009): 99–106. https://doi.org/10.1111/j.1750-2659.2009.00080.x.

Armati, Marco, ed. Urban Green Belts in the Twenty-First Century. London: Ashgate, 2008.

Autengruber, Peter. Die Wiener Kleingärten: Von den Anfängen bis zur Gegenwart. Wien: Promedia, 2018.

Breiling, Meinhard, and Gisa Ruland. "The Vienna Green Belt: From Localised Protection to a Regional Concept." In Urban Green Belts in the Twenty-First Century. Edited by Marco Armati, 167–83. London: Ashgate, 2008.

Chang, Tu-Hsuan, Yu-Chin Chen, Wei-Yu Chen, Chun-Yu Chen, Wei-Yun Hsu, Yun Chou, and Yi-Hsin Chang. "Weight Gain Associated with COVID-19 Lockdown in Children and Adolescents: A Systematic Review and Meta-Analysis." Nutrients 13, no. 10 (2021). https://doi.org/10.3390/nu13103668.

Czech, Herwig. "Joseph II. Und Die Erste Wiener Medizinische Schule." Accessed March 31, 2020. https://magazin.wienmuseum.at/joseph-ii-und-die-erste-wiener-medizinische-schule.

Dietrich-Daum, Elisabeth. Die „Wiener Krankheit": Eine Sozialgeschichte der Tuberkulose in Österreich. Sozial- und Wirtschaftshistorische Studien Bd. 32. Wien, München: Verlag für Geschichte und Politik; Oldenbourg-Wissenschaftsverlag, 2007.

Gugerell, Katharina, and Stefan Netsch. "Reflection on the Austrian Newspaper Coverage of the Role and Relevance of Urban Open-and Green-Spaces in Vienna During the First COVID-19 Lockdown in 2020." disP – The Planning Review 56, no. 4 (2020): 54–63. https://doi.org/10.1080/02513625.2020.1906051.

Häberlin, Udo, Gerlinde Mückstein, Nils Peters, Gregor Stratil-Sauer, Johannes Suitner, Tobias Troger, and Maria Wasserburger. "Corona: Die Rolle Der Stadtplanung Für Die Krisenbewältigung Am Beispiel Wien." REAL CORP, 2020, 1271–80.

Haider, Edgard. Wien 1918: Agonie Der Kaiserstadt. Wien, Köln, Weimar: Böhlau, 2018.

Holmberg, Martin. Pandemier Och Epidemier – Från Kolera till Covid-19 I Ett Tvärvetenskapligt Perspektiv. 2nd ed. Studentlitteratur AB, 2020.

Hu, Dalong, Bin Liu, Lu Feng, Peng Ding, Xi Guo, Min Wang, Boyang Cao, Peter R. Reeves, and Lei Wang. "Origins of the Current Seventh Cholera Pandemic." Proceedings of the National Academy of Sciences of the United States of America 113, no. 48 (2016): E7730-E7739. https://doi.org/10.1073/pnas.1608732113.

Ichner, Bernhard. "Wien Gehört zu den grünsten Metropolen Europas." Kurier, May 2, 2019. https://kurier.at/chronik/wien/wien-gehoert-zu-den-gruensten-metropolen-europas/400480591.

Koszteczky, Gertraud. "Die Geschichte der Wiener Grünflächen im Zusammenhang mit dem sozialen Wandel ihrer BenützerInnen." Dissertation, Universtiät Wien, 2007.

Madner, Martina. "Was Zu Ostern (Nicht) Erlaubt ist." Wiener Zeitung. Accessed April 1, 2021. https://www.wienerzeitung.at/nachrichten/politik/oesterreich/2098706-Was-zu-Ostern-nicht-erlaubt-ist.html.

Oscilowicz, Emilia. "Policy and Planning Toolkit for Urban Green Justice." Barcelona Laboratory for Urban Environmental Justice and Sustainability.

Pataki, Diane E., Margaret M. Carreiro, Jennifer Cherrier, Nancy E. Grulke, Viniece Jennings, Stephanie Pincetl, Richard V. Pouyat, Thomas H. Whitlow, and Wayne C. Zipperer. "Coupling Biogeochemical Cycles in Urban Environments: Ecosystem Services, Green Solutions, and Misconceptions." Frontiers in Ecology and the Environment 9, no. 1 (2011): 27–36. https://doi.org/10.1890/090220.

Rosenberg, Charles E. Explaining Epidemics and Other Studies in the History of Medicine. Cambridge: Cambridge University Press, 1992. https://doi.org/10.1017/CBO9780511666865.

Schmidbauer, Julia. ",Zweiter Lockdown – Diese Corona-Regeln gelten jetzt in Österreich." Mein Bezirk, November 17, 2020. https://www.meinbezirk.at/c-politik/diese-corona-regeln-gelten-jetzt-in-oesterreich_a4351529.

Seydl, Robert. "Visions & New Beginnings – 150 Years of the Vienna World's Fair." Vienna, Intl. 124.

Spreeuwenberg, Peter, Madelon Kroneman, and John Paget. "Reassessing the Global Mortality Burden of the 1918 Influenza Pandemic." American journal of epidemiology 187, no. 12 (2018): 2561–67. https://doi.org/10.1093/aje/kwy191.

Stadt Wien. "Stadtentwicklungsplan STEP 2035 – Urban Development Plan 2035." Accessed May 12, 2023. https://www.wien.gv.at/stadtentwicklung/strategien/step/step2035/.

Stadt Wien. "Grünflächen nach Nutzungsklassen und Bezirken 2021." https://www.wien.gv.at/statistik/lebensraum/tabellen/gruenflaechen-bez.html.

Stadt Wien, Baupolizei. "Informationsblatt für Bauvorhaben im Kleingartengebiet."

Stadt Wien, MA18. "Urban Development Plan Vienna STEP 2025." 2014.

Stadt Wien, Stadtentwicklung und Stadtplanung. "Green and Open Spaces – Thematic Concept." 2015.

Suttinger, Daniel. "Wienn in Österreich/Auff Ihro Keyserliche Mayest: Allergnädigsten Befehing/in Grundt Gelegt Und in Gegenwärtigen Riß Verfertiget." Stadtplan Anno 1684. https://www.wien.gv.at/actaproweb2/benutzung/image.xhtml?id=RYNtWiQTRldd50I2WlVEduM0+8OkdD4Jp25sfgC2ACs1.

Tansil, Donna, Christian Plecak, Karolina Taczanowska, and Alexandra Jiricka-Pürrer. "Experience Them, Love Them, Protect Them-Has the COVID-19 Pandemic Changed People's Perception of Urban and Suburban Green Spaces and Their Conservation Targets?" Environmental management 70, no. 6 (2022): 1004-22. https://doi.org/10.1007/s00267-022-01721-9.

Teleky, Ludwig. "Die Sterblichkeit an Tuberkulose in Österreich 1873-1904." Statistische Monatsschrift, 1906, 145.

Velimirovic, Boris, and Helga Velimirovic. "Plague in Vienna." Reviews of Infectious Diseases 11, no. 5 (1989): 808-26. http://www.jstor.org/stable/4455344.

Weigl, Andreas. "Demographischer Wandel und Modernisierung in Wien, 1700 bis 1999." 2003.

Weigl, Andreas. "Epidemien Statistik - Lieferung 8, Historischer Atlas der Stadt Wien." 2020.

Weihsmann, Helmut. Das Rote Wien: Sozialdemokratische Architektur und Kommunalpolitik 1919-1934. 2nd ed. Wien: Promedia.

Winterer, Matthias. "In der Hitze der Stadt." Wiener Zeitung, June 19, 2022.

Winterer, Matthias. "Zu wenig Grün für alle." Wiener Zeitung, March 21, 2023.

Urban Green Space Planning for New Work Styles in the Post-Pandemic Era[1]

Takahiro Yamazaki, Akiko Iida, Kimihiro Hino,
Akito Murayama, U Hiroi, Toru Terada, Hideki Koizumi,
Makoto Yokohari

Introduction

Background and objectives

On 30 January 2020, the World Health Organisation (WHO) declared an international public health emergency due to the coronavirus disease 2019 (COVID-19) pandemic[2]. Governments around the world implemented quarantine measures to minimise the chances of human-to-human contact[3]. Workers who commuted to the central business district almost every day were strongly urged to switch to telecommuting. Most public meeting facilities frequented by older adults, and schools attended by children were temporarily closed. With the exception of essential workers, city dwellers were forced to stay home, regardless of their lifestyle. In cities around the world, lifestyles changed drastically.

Tokyo, Japan, has one of the largest populations in the world, with people living together in a very dense environment. Thus, the governor of Tokyo encouraged behaviour that avoids the 3Cs (closed spaces, crowded places, and

---

[1] The content of this chapter is based on the following paper: Yamazaki, Takahiro, Akiko Iida, Kimihiro Hino, Akito Murayama, U Hiroi, Toru Terada, Hideki Koizumi, and Makoto Yokohari, "Use of Urban Green Spaces in the Context of Lifestyle Changes during the COVID-19 Pandemic in Tokyo."
[2] World Health Organization, "Statement on the Second Meeting of the International Health Regulations (2005) Emergency Committee Regarding the Outbreak of Novel Coronavirus (2019-nCoV)."
[3] Hale et al., "Variation in Government Responses to COVID-19, Version 7.0."

close-contact settings) to reduce the spread of the first wave of COVID-19[4]. For example, trains in Tokyo are very congested compared with other cities due to the city's urban structure, with functions concentrated in the city centre; therefore, to avoid the 3Cs on trains, the governor set a goal of reducing the number of people commuting to work by 70%. To achieve this goal, many companies had to adopt telecommuting systems[5]. Even before the pandemic, Tokyo had already been regarded as a workaholic city. Working hours and commuting time were long, and time spent on leisure was short, resulting in a work–life balance that had been rated poor compared to cities in other countries[6]. Therefore, the rapid spread of telecommuting due to the pandemic should have resulted in a drastic shift in work styles[7]. The transformation of telecommuting as a common work style option is also expected to contribute to an improved work–life balance in Tokyo. Another characteristic of Tokyo is its high aging rate. At 51%, Japan has the world's highest percentage of older adults aged 65 and above as a percentage of its population aged 20 and over, as of 2019[8]. The spread of COVID-19 among older adults, who are at a high risk of contracting severe disease, would have pressured the limited healthcare supply system[9]. Accordingly, the closing of public meeting facilities that tended to be frequented by older adults was undertaken as a priority quarantine measure for the first wave of COVID-19. The other major quarantine measure, as implemented in other countries, was the closure of educational institutions from nursery schools to universities[10]. Hence, workers, older adults, and children and their families had to make drastic changes in their lifestyles.

Urban green spaces (UGS) are likely to be valuable places for individuals who are virtually forced to live in and around their homes. These places allow people to exercise and rest without worrying about the 3Cs, whereas refraining from going out causes problems of lack of exercise and stress accumulation. In fact, the number of people using UGS seems to have increased during the pandemic[11], except in countries that had strong lockdowns in place during the

---

[4] Tokyo Metropolitan Government, "Message to the People of Tokyo: Refrain from Going Out at Night (Message from the Governor)."
[5] Karako et al., "Shifting Workstyle to Teleworking as a New Normal in Face of COVID-19: Analysis with the Model Introducing Intercity Movement and Behavioral Pattern."
[6] Organisation for Economic Co-Operation and Development, "Work-Life Balance."
[7] Tokyo Metropolitan Government, "Results of the Urgent Survey about Telework Introduction Rate."
[8] United Nations, Department of Economic and Social Affairs, Population Division, "World Population Ageing 2019: Highlights (ST/ESA/SER.A/430)."
[9] Verity et al., "Estimates of the Severity of Coronavirus Disease 2019: A Model-Based Analysis."
[10] Mathieu et al., "OurWorld in Data."
[11] Venter et al., "Urban Nature in a Time of Crisis: Recreational Use of Green Space Increases During the COVID-19 Outbreak in Oslo, Norway."

pandemic[12]. In megacities, in particular, houses, gardens, and balconies are usually small. A survey in Europe and South America found that city residents who spent the lockdown period in smaller houses had a lower sense of well-being[13]. It seems that UGS were essential places of exercise and rest for megacity residents during the pandemic. However, it has been reported that there are many people whose use of UGS decreases as well as those whose use of UGS increases, even if the use of UGS is not restricted[14]. Therefore, it is important to understand how and by whom UGS were used and valued by megacity residents during the COVID-19 pandemic to enhance urban resilience.

The purpose of this study was to clarify the relationship between individuals' personal characteristics and the use of UGS during the COVID-19 pandemic in Tokyo. Specifically, this study focused on telecommuters, older adults, and families with children, whose lifestyle may have been drastically changed due to the COVID-19 pandemic. The analysis focused on whether UGS were used, based on each type of UGS, and how users evaluated and perceived the use of UGS. Based on the results, this study discusses points that should be considered for planning UGS in the post-COVID-19 society.

Previous surveys

Many studies have discussed the health and well-being effects of UGS[15,16,17,18,19,20,21,22]. Bedimo-Rung et al.[23] proposed a model of the process by which UGS can

---

[12] Geng et al., "Impacts of COVID-19 Pandemic on Urban Park Visitation: A Global Analysis."
[13] Pérez-Urrestarazu et al., "Particularities of Having Plants at Home During the Confinement Due to the COVID-19 Pandemic."
[14] Berdejo-Espinola et al., "Urban Green Space Use During a Time of Stress: A Case Study During the COVID-19 Pandemic in Brisbane, Australia."
[15] Takano, Nakamura and Watanabe, "Urban Residential Environments and Senior Citizens' Longevity in Megacity Areas: The Importance of Walkable Green Spaces."
[16] Ward Thomson et al., "More Green Space Is Linked to Less Stress in Deprived Communities: Evidence from Salivary Cortisol Patterns."
[17] Kardan et al., "Neighborhood Greenspace and Health in a Large Urban Center."
[18] Cox et al., "Doses of Neighborhood Nature: The Benefits for Mental Health of Living with Nature."
[19] Lafortezza et al., "Benefits and Well-Being Perceived by People Visiting Green Spaces in Periods of Heat Stress."
[20] Korpela et al., "Analyzing the Mediators Between Nature-Based Outdoor Recreation and Emotional Well-Being."
[21] Grilli, Mohan and Curtis, "Public Park Attributes, Park Visits, and Associated Health Status."
[22] Shanahan et al., "Health benefits from nature experiences depend on dose."
[23] Bedimo-Rung et al., "The Significance of Parks to Physical Activity and Public Health: A Conceptual Model."

properly exert these effects[24]. According to the model, two factors influence the improvement of health and well-being through the use of UGS: the characteristics of the user and the characteristics of the UGS. In other words, considering user characteristics is as important as considering spatial characteristics if urban planners want to increase the benefits of UGS.

Several studies have analysed the relationship between UGS and user characteristics[25,26]. Age is frequently discussed as a personal attribute that strongly influences the use of UGS. Older adults[27,28,29,30] and younger people[31,32,33] tend to use UGS more. Among young people, families with children have particularly high rates of using UGS.[34,35,36,37] The influence of gender has also been noted. Depending on the study, there appear to be higher rates of utilisation for

---

[24] Bedimo-Rung, Mowen and Cohen, "The Significance of Parks to Physical Activity and Public Health: A Conceptual Model."
[25] Kaczynski and Henderson, "Environmental Correlates of Physical Activity: A Review of Evidence About Parks and Recreation."
[26] Kloek et al., "Shifting Workstyle to Teleworking as a New Normal in Face of COVID-19: Analysis with the Model Introducing Intercity Movement and Behavioral Pattern."
[27] Schipperijn et al., "Factors Influencing the Use of Green Space: Results from a Danish National Representative Survey."
[28] Schipperijn et al., "Influences on the Use of Urban Green Space – a Case Study in Odense, Denmark."
[29] Jim and Chen, "Recreation-amenity Use and Contingent Valuation of Urban Greenspaces in Guangzhou, China."
[30] Wong, "Urban Park Visiting Habits and Leisure Activities of Residents in Hong Kong, China."
[31] Boyd et al., "Who Doesn't Visit Natural Environments for Recreation and Why: A Population Representative Analysis of Spatial, Individual and Temporal Factors Among Adults in England."
[32] Sanesi and Chiarello, "Residents and Urban Green Spaces: The Case of Bari."
[33] Sreetheran, "Exploring the Urban Park Use, Preference and Behaviours Among the Residents of Kuala Lumpur, Malaysia."
[34] Schipperijn et al., "Influences on the Use of Urban Green Space – a Case Study in Odense, Denmark."
[35] Jim and Chen, "Recreation-amenity Use and Contingent Valuation of Urban Greenspaces in Guangzhou, China."
[36] Wong, "Urban Park Visiting Habits and Leisure Activities of Residents in Hong Kong, China."
[37] Boyd et al., "Who Doesn't Visit Natural Environments for Recreation and Why: A Population Representative Analysis of Spatial, Individual and Temporal Factors Among Adults in England."

males[38,39] as well as females[40]. Some studies have also mentioned the influence of race[41]. Moreover, several studies have pointed to the impact of living characteristics on the use of UGS. Those with roommates[42,43], dogs[44], and those living in the suburbs[45] have been found to be more likely to use UGS. One study has discussed work styles in relation to using UGS. It appears that people use UGS more when they are not working full-time[46]. Given the increase in the number of telecommuters due to the COVID-19 pandemic, it is important to understand how these changes in work style have affected the use of UGS.

Several pioneering studies have targeted the use of UGS during the COVID-19 pandemic. Geng et al.[47] analysed the trends and determinants of UGS visitation by country using the Google COVID-19 Community Mobility Report for 48 countries from 16 February to 26 May, 2020. Ugolini et al.[48] conducted an online survey between 12 April and 4 May, 2020, in six countries in Europe and the Middle East to compare the use and perception of UGS before and after the pandemic by country. These two international comparative studies concluded that trends in the use of UGS were largely influenced by the stringency of government quarantine policies. In addition to global studies, some case studies have been conducted on specific cities or nations to examine

---

[38] Boyd et al., "Who Doesn't Visit Natural Environments for Recreation and Why: A Population Representative Analysis of Spatial, Individual and Temporal Factors Among Adults in England."

[39] Wright Wendel, Zarger, and Mihelcic, "Accessibility and Usability: Green Space Preferences, Perceptions, and Barriers in a Rapidly Urbanizing City in Latin America."

[40] Sang et al., "The Effects of Naturalness, Gender, and Age on How Urban Green Space Is Perceived and Used."

[41] Boyd et al., "Who Doesn't Visit Natural Environments for Recreation and Why: A Population Representative Analysis of Spatial, Individual and Temporal Factors Among Adults in England."

[42] Boyd et al., "Who Doesn't Visit Natural Environments for Recreation and Why: A Population Representative Analysis of Spatial, Individual and Temporal Factors Among Adults in England."

[43] Sanesi and Chiarello, "Residents and Urban Green Spaces: The Case of Bari."

[44] Schipperijn et al., "Influences on the Use of Urban Green Space – a Case Study in Odense, Denmark."

[45] Sanesi and Chiarello, "Residents and Urban Green Spaces: The Case of Bari."

[46] Boyd et al., "Who Doesn't Visit Natural Environments for Recreation and Why: A Population Representative Analysis of Spatial, Individual and Temporal Factors Among Adults in England."

[47] Geng et al., "Impacts of COVID-19 Pandemic on Urban Park Visitation: A Global Analysis."

[48] Ugolini et al., "Effects of the COVID-19 Pandemic on the Use and Perceptions of Urban Green Space: An International Exploratory Study."

trends in the use of UGS. Venter et al.[49] compared the number of users of UGS before and during the pandemic through mobile data analysis in the city of Oslo, Norway, and concluded that the number of users of UGS increased by 291 % during the pandemic. Meanwhile, Berdejo-Espinola et al.[50] showed that not all city residents increased their frequency of UGS use. A questionnaire examining the frequency of UGS use in Brisbane, Australia, during and before the country's periods of mobility restrictions showed that 26 % of respondents used UGS less, while 36 % used them more. The study shows that the frequency of use tended to decrease with age. Xie et al.[51] conducted an online survey of park users in Chengdu, China, from 1 April to 5 April 2020, to analyse the health and well-being benefits of UGS. It appears that users of UGS were able to improve their physical health and meet their social interaction needs during the pandemic. The results of an online survey conducted in Mexico City, Mexico by Huerta and Utomo[52] similarly showed that the use of UGS during the pandemic contributed to improved subjective well-being among individuals. Poortinga et al.[53] analysed a Welsh government survey on the health of the UK Welsh population and found that the use of UGS contributed to people's improved subjective well-being and sense of health during the pandemic, regardless of age or gender.

Three studies of the Tokyo metropolitan area during the pandemic mention UGS use. Lu et al.[54] analysed online posts on the photo-sharing social media networking service Instagram from four Asian cities, including Tokyo, and found that people preferred parks that were close to the city centre, large in size, and rich in nature. Soga et al.[55] conducted an online survey in Tokyo and found that people were more likely to use green spaces if they had a view of greenery from their homes. Hino and Asami[56] analysed the relationship

---

[49] Venter et al., "Urban Nature in a Time of Crisis: Recreational Use of Green Space Increases During the COVID-19 Outbreak in Oslo, Norway."

[50] Berdejo-Espinola et al., "Urban Green Space Use During a Time of Stress: A Case Study During the COVID-19 Pandemic in Brisbane, Australia."

[51] Xie et al., "Urban Parks as Green Buffers During the COVID-19 Pandemic."

[52] Mayen, Huerta and Utomo, "Evaluating the Association Between Urban Green Spaces and Subjective Well-Being in Mexico City During the COVID-19 Pandemic."

[53] Poortinga, "The Role of Perceived Public and Private Green Space in Subjective Health and Wellbeing During and After the First Peak of the COVID-19 Outbreak."

[54] Lu, "Escaping to Nature During a Pandemic: A Natural Experiment in Asian Cities During the COVID-19 Pandemic with Big Social Media Data."

[55] Soga et al., "A Room with a Green View: The Importance of Nearby Nature for Mental Health During the COVID-19 Pandemic."

[56] Hino and Asami, "Change in Walking Steps and Association with Built Environments During the COVID-19 State of Emergency: A Longitudinal Comparison with the First Half of 2019 in Yokohama, Japan."

between the number of steps taken in a day and the location of residence in Yokohama City, which is within the Tokyo metropolitan area, and compared results during and before the pandemic. Consequently, while the number of steps was found to have decreased significantly in densely populated areas, the number of steps did not decrease as much when the distance to a large UGS was close. For older women in particular, the decrease in steps was found to be mitigated when they lived near a large park. These studies suggest that the use of UGS had been important in Tokyo during the pandemic. However, there have been limited studies on UGS during the pandemic that take into account the characteristics of the users, even though their lifestyles have been drastically changed by the COVID-19 pandemic.

Methods

Characteristics of the survey area and the pandemic period

In Japan, a state of emergency was declared on 7 April, 2020, in response to the initial wave of COVID-19. The declaration of a state of emergency is the most severe measure that the Japanese government can take under the law. In Tokyo, the state of emergency was in effect for about 1.5 months until 25 May, when the medical system began to improve.

Residents of Tokyo during this emergency period were asked by the government to voluntarily refrain from leaving their homes unnecessarily[57]. For example, they were asked to reduce the number of times they commuted to work or school and refrain from holding or participating in events. However, there was no obligation to record one's outings using healthcare mobile applications to enable contact tracing, nor was there any penalty for going out. In addition, the government informed that "people can go out when it is necessary to maintain their lives, such as going to medical institutions, shopping for daily necessities, going to essential workplaces, and walking or jogging to maintain their health"[58]. In other words, Japanese quarantine measures were not as strict as lockdowns in Western countries[59,60]. Therefore, UGS around the home, which are easy to use and avoid the 3Cs, would have been valuable

---

[57] Tashiro and Shaw, "COVID-19 Pandemic Response in Japan: What Is Behind the Initial Flattening of the Curve?"

[58] Cabinet Secretariat, Government of Japan, "About the New Influenza Special Measures Act, COVID-19 Information and Resources."

[59] Tashiro and Shaw, "COVID-19 Pandemic Response in Japan: What Is Behind the Initial Flattening of the Curve?"

[60] Hale and Webster, "Oxford Covid-19 Government Response Tracker."

places for exercise and rest during the emergency period. In fact, most of the UGS in Tokyo, whether publicly or privately owned, could be used during the emergency period as long as physical distancing was maintained. However, parking lots and stands were closed, and some gated UGS, such as gardens and university campuses were closed as well. During this period, Tokyo had only one rainy day per week, and the maximum temperature ranged from 15° C to 25° C, making it easy to spend time outdoors.

Focusing on UGS in Tokyo, there is a lack of parks owned by the local government; however, there is a relative abundance of various types of UGS owned by individuals and organisations. Urban parks are about 5.7 m2 per capita as of 2020[61], which is a very low ratio when compared to that of other large cities. However, while the number of urban parks may be insufficient, privately owned UGS exist to a certain extent in Tokyo. For example, there are 4327 temple and shrine sites in Tokyo[62], compared to 8287 urban parks[63].

Study questionnaire

A questionnaire survey was conducted using the platform provided by Macromill, Inc. (Tokyo, Japan), an online research company. A total of 3096 people aged 20 and above living in Tokyo responded to the questionnaire. The number of respondents was adjusted while recruiting so that they would be evenly distributed across age groups (those in their 20s, 30s, 40s, 50s, 60s, and 70s and above) and residing areas (Tokyo special wards and Tama suburban cities). The survey was conducted between 4 June and 8 June 2020, after the end of the first declaration of state of emergency by the national government.

The questions in the questionnaire survey comprised three main categories. The first category included questions on personal information, such as gender, age, co-residents, residential area, work style during the emergency period, and changes in work hours during the emergency period. The second set of questions captured the use of UGS. For each of the six types of UGS (small parks and plazas, large parks and plazas, greenways and riverbeds, urban forests, temple and shrine grounds, and urban farmlands) (Fig. 1), the survey asked whether the respondents used them, and whether they had been using those UGS only recently, i.e., were new users of the UGS. The third set of questions focused on the evaluations and perceptions of the users of UGS. The following

---

[61] Bureau of Construction, Tokyo Metropolitan Government, "Parks in Tokyo."
[62] Agency for Cultural Affairs, Government of Japan, "Religious Statistics Database 2020."
[63] Bureau of Construction, Tokyo Metropolitan Government, "Urban Green Space Database 2020."

eight items were assessed using a five-point scale ("strongly agree", "agree", "neutral", "disagree", and "strongly disagree"): I felt satisfied with exercising and resting in the UGS; I felt relieved of anxiety and stress; I felt less lonely; I felt connected to others in a relaxed way; I was able to maintain a sufficient physical distance in the UGS; I was able to use the UGS without worrying about the eyes around me; It was an opportunity for me to become aware of the existence of nature around me that I had not noticed before; It was an opportunity for me to become aware of the good qualities of the area where I live.

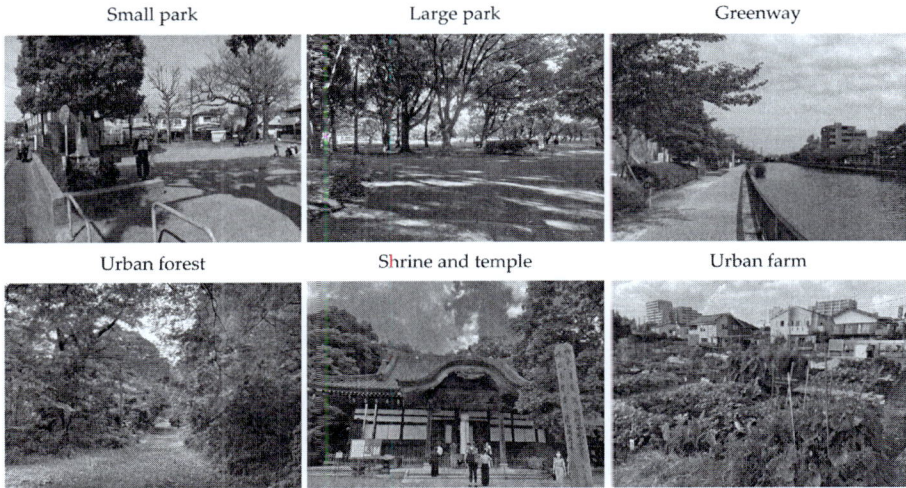

Fig. 1: Urban green space types in Tokyo (Illustration: Takahiro Yamazaki, Akiko Iida, Kimihiro Hino, Akito Murayama, U Hiroi, Toru Terada, Hideki Koizumi, Makoto Yokohari)

Statistical analysis methods

A binomial logistic regression analysis was conducted using three models (Table A1). Model 1 was used to determine whether UGS were used during the emergency period and whether there were new users of UGS. Model 2 determined whether UGS were used based on the type of UGS. Model 3 focused on the evaluations and perceptions of the use of UGS. In Model 3, responses on a five-point scale were categorised into binary variables with "1" for "strongly agree" or "agree" and "0" for other options.

The explanatory variables were respondents' personal characteristics. The main target groups were telecommuters, older adults, and families with children, whose lifestyles are expected to have been significantly affected by the pandemic. As control factors, the characteristics of the users of UGS, which have been pointed out in previous studies, were added (Table A2); these characteristics were: being male, having a roommate, living in the suburbs, and owning a dog. In addition, a previous study has discussed the relationship between full-time work and use of UGS[64]. Given the strong influence of the pandemic on work hours, we added non-workers and reduced worktime as control factors. Nine explanatory variables were used (Table A3). According to Peduzzi et al. (1996), the event per variables should be less than 10[65]. For this reason, urban farmland (2F) with less than 90 respondents was excluded from the regression analysis in this study.

A sample of 3085 valid responses was obtained by selecting those who responded to all the variables used in the analysis. The significance level was set at $p < 0.05$. R version 4.0.2 was used for analysis.

Ethical considerations

This survey underwent an ethical review by the University of Tokyo, and preparations were made to ensure that the respondents are given enough consideration (approval number: KE20-8). Only those researchers who had completed the University of Tokyo's ethics course were involved in the storing and analysing of data. All survey respondents consented to participate in Macromill's anonymous online survey. There was a financial incentive for respondents. All respondents understood the purpose of the survey and were informed of their right to withdraw anytime during the survey.

Results

General information of the respondents

The explanatory variables generated from the personal attributes of the 3085 respondents revealed that telecommuters, older adults, and families with children

---

[64] Boyd et al., "Who Doesn't Visit Natural Environments for Recreation and Why: A Population Representative Analysis of Spatial, Individual and Temporal Factors Among Adults in England."

[65] Peduzzi et al., "A Simulation Study of the Number of Events Per Variable in Logistic Regression Analysis."

made up 37%, 23%, and 14% of the respondents, respectively. In addition, 53% of the respondents were male. In terms of housing, 75% lived with someone, and 6% owned a dog (Table A3).

While 37% of the respondents were telecommuters, 30% were workers who commuted physically, and the remaining 33% did not work. Among the telecommuters, 90% were first-time home workers during the emergency period. Approximately 60% of the telecommuters did not commute at all, while approximately 40% commuted a few days a week. During the emergency period, 34% of telecommuters and 39% of commuters worked fewer hours than usual (Table A4).

		Total		Telecommuter		Older Adult		Family with children	
		n	%	n	%	n	%	n	%
	Total (all)	3085	100%	1132	100%	708	100	434	100
1A	Users of UGS	1423	46%	551	49%	389	55%	263	61%
1B	New users of UGS	300	10%	141	12%	62	9%	50	12%
2A	Small park users	751	24%	286	25%	195	28%	204	47%
2B	Large park users	594	19%	260	23%	162	23%	131	30%
2C	Greenway users	926	30%	371	33%	240	34%	150	35%
2D	Urban forest users	260	3%	102	9%	92	13%	47	11%
2E	Temple and/or shrine users	283	9%	125	11%	77	11%	38	9%
2F	Urban farmland users	65	2%	40	4%	11	2%	12	3%
	Total (users of UGS)	1423	46%	551	49%	389	55%	263	61%
3A	Felt satisfied with UGS	871	61%	367	67%	240	62%	168	64%
3B	Useful for stress relief	863	61%	358	65%	230	59%	159	60%
3C	Reduced loneliness	376	26%	166	30%	87	22%	86	33%
3D	Felt a connection with others	342	24%	130	24%	98	25%	86	33%
3E	Distancing can be maintained	945	66%	349	63%	311	80%	168	64%
3F	Able to use UGS without being self-conscious	883	62%	341	62%	300	77%	138	52%
3G	Noticed nature in close proximity	641	45%	283	51%	169	43%	127	48%
3H	Noticed positive aspects of my neighbourhood	720	51%	315	57%	203	52%	145	55%
UGS: urban green space									

Table 1: Use of UGS by groups

General results

This section summarises the simple tabulation of the results of the questionnaire responses that were treated as objective variables in Models 1 through 3 (Table 1). First, 46% of the respondents used UGS. During the emergency period, the government allowed outdoor exercise, but less than half of the respondents actually used UGS. Moreover, 10% of respondents started using UGS during the emergency period. In this sense, the pandemic may have been an opportunity for them to use UGS that they had not used recently. Next, focusing on the type of UGS used, most people used greenways and riverbeds (30%), followed by small parks (24%) and large parks (19%). Publicly owned UGS were the most commonly used; however, there were also a certain number of users of temple and shrine land (9%), urban forest land (8%), and urban farmland (2%), most of which are privately owned.

With regard to the respondents' evaluations and perceptions of UGS (n = 1423), 61% of the users of UGS seemed to be satisfied with their exercise and rest in the UGS. In terms of the function of UGS, relatively more people (61%) felt that UGS had a function of relieving anxiety and stress, while a lesser proportion of them were of the view that UGS could relieve loneliness (26%) or help them feel connected to others (24%). This may be due in part to the fact that people refrained from communicating when using UGS during the emergency

period. Indeed, 66% of the respondents perceived that they were able to use the UGS while maintaining physical distance. Finally, as a result of using the UGS, 45% of the respondents became aware of the surrounding nature, and 51% realised the goodness of the community.

Model 1: Use of UGS

The relationship between the use of UGS and user characteristics was analysed using binomial logistic regression (Table 2). The results showed that telecommuters (odds ratio [OR] = 1.489, $p < 0.001$), older adults (OR = 1.824, $p < 0.001$), and families with children (OR = 2.329, $p < 0.001$) often used UGS at a highly significant level (Model 1A). Other factors such as owning a dog (OR = 1.639, $p = 0.001$), being male (OR = 1.165, $p = 0.051$), and not working (OR = 1.218, $p = 0.054$) were also related to the use of UGS. In contrast to previous studies, living with someone or living in the suburbs was found to be unlikely to affect the use of UGS in Tokyo during the emergency period. Telecommuters (OR = 1.535, $p = 0.004$) and women (OR = 1.815, $p < 0.001$) were more likely to be new users of UGS during the emergency period (Model 1B). The odds ratio for telecommuters was larger than that for older adults and families with children, suggesting that the pandemic was an opportunity for them to commence the use of UGS. Additionally, based on the analysis that adjusted for the decreased worktime, the tendency of the new use of UGS by telecommuters was revealed. In other words, telecommuting may have accelerated the new use of UGS, regardless of whether work hours increased or decreased.

	Model 1A				Model 1B			
	Users of UGS				New Users of UGS			
	Odds Ratio	Std. Error	p-Value		Odds Ratio	Std. Error	p-Value	
Intercept	0.427	0.113	0.000	***	0.118	0.181	0.000	***
Telecommuter	1.489	0.092	0.000	***	1.535	0.148	0.004	**
Older adult	1.824	0.104	0.000	***	1.415	0.179	0.052	
Family with children	2.329	0.114	0.000	***	1.235	0.178	0.237	
Male	1.165	0.078	0.051		0.551	0.131	0.000	***
Living with someone	1.096	0.090	0.309		0.939	0.148	0.669	
Dog owner	1.639	0.155	0.001	**	0.523	0.333	0.052	
Living in suburbs	1.057	0.075	0.457		1.125	0.124	0.344	
Not worker	1.218	0.102	0.054		0.729	0.181	0.081	
Decreased worktime	1.045	0.081	0.583		1.088	0.131	0.521	

UGS: urban green space.* p < 0.05; ** p < 0.01; *** p < 0.001.

Table 2. Use of UGS and user characteristics (Model 1)

Model 2: Use of UGS type

The relationship between the use of the five types of UGS and user characteristics was analysed using binomial logistic regression (Table 3). The results showed that telecommuters, older adults, and families with children commonly used large parks, greenways, and urban forests significantly more (Models 2B-D). Greenways for telecommuters (OR = 1.541, p < 0.001), large parks for families with children (OR = 2.382, p < 0.001), and urban forests for older adults (OR = 1.888, p < 0.001) had relatively large odds ratios. Furthermore, older adults (OR = 1.563, p < 0.001) and families with children (OR = 4.534, p < 0.001) significantly used small parks more often, whereas telecommuters did not (Model 2A). In contrast, telecommuters significantly used temple and shrine areas more often (OR = 1.699, p = 0.001), but older adults and families with children did not (Model 2E).

	Model 2A				Model 2B			
	Small Park				Large Park			
	Odds Ratio	Std. Error	p-Value		Odds Ratio	Std. Error	p-Value	
Intercept	0.183	0.137	0.000	***	0.098	0.155	0.000	***
Telecommuter	1.192	0.109	0.108		1.713	0.118	0.000	***
Older adult	1.563	0.121	0.000	***	1.589	0.130	0.000	***
Family with children	4.534	0.122	0.000	***	2.382	0.130	0.000	***
Male	1.530	0.095	0.000	***	1.437	0.101	0.000	***
Living with someone	0.892	0.110	0.297		1.271	0.122	0.050	
Dog owner	1.628	0.171	0.004	**	1.614	0.179	0.007	**
Living in suburbs	0.826	0.088	0.029	*	0.834	0.094	0.054	
Not worker	1.155	0.121	0.236		1.199	0.135	0.177	
Decreased worktime	0.960	0.096	0.667		1.089	0.102	0.402	
UGS: urban green space. * p ≤ 0.05; ** p ≤ 0.01; *** p ≤ 0.001								

Table 3: Use of UGS type and user characteristics (Model 2)

	Model 2C				Model 2D				Model 2E			
	Greenway				Urban Forest				Shrine and Temple			
	Odds Ratio	Std. Error	p-Value		Odds Ratio	Std. Error	p-Value		Odds Ratio	Std. Error	p-Value	
Intercept	0.229	0.125	0.000	***	0.016	0.248	0.000	***	0.061	0.202	0.000	***
Telecommuter	1.541	0.100	0.000	***	1.554	0.173	0.011	*	1.699	0.162	0.001	**
Older adult	1.335	0.111	0.009	**	1.888	0.177	0.000	***	1.243	0.172	0.207	
Family with children	1.330	0.118	0.016	*	1.679	0.191	0.007	**	1.022	0.196	0.914	
Male	1.053	0.085	0.540		1.812	0.151	0.000	***	1.276	0.135	0.071	
Living with someone	1.090	0.099	0.381		1.318	0.182	0.130		1.100	0.155	0.540	
Dog owner	1.256	0.161	0.157		1.018	0.276	0.949		0.971	0.272	0.915	
Living in suburbs	1.231	0.080	0.009	**	2.789	0.146	0.000	***	0.735	0.128	0.016	*
Not worker	1.308	0.111	0.016	*	1.240	0.191	0.260		1.389	0.185	0.076	
Decreased worktime	1.171	0.086	0.066		1.076	0.147	0.619		1.192	0.135	0.194	
UGS: urban green space. * p ≤ 0.05; ** p ≤ 0.01; *** p ≤ 0.001												

Table 3: Use of UGS type and user characteristics (Model 2)

Model 3: Evaluation of use of UGS

The relationship between the characteristics of users of UGS and their evaluations and perceptions of UGS was analysed using binomial logistic regression (Table 4). First, telecommuters were found to be relatively satisfied with their use of UGS (OR = 1.448, p = 0.005) (Model 3A). In addition, while more than 60% of UGS users during the emergency period appreciated the relief from anxiety and stress through using UGS, telecommuters were more likely to rate it (OR = 1.259, p = 0.082) (Model 3B). Next, older adults (OR = 1.507, p = 0.019) and families with children (OR = 1.895, p < 0.001) commonly felt more connected to others by using UGS (Model 3D). In particular, older adults seemed to be able to use the UGS without worrying about others (OR = 2.020, p < 0.001) and keeping their distance from others (OR = 2.176, p < 0.001) (Models 3E and 3F). Families with children appeared to have appreciated the relief from loneliness made possible by their use of UGS (OR = 1.335, p = 0.077) (Model 3C). Finally, telecommuters (OR = 1.506, p = 0.003) and older adults (OR = 1.570, p = 0.003) shared the tendency to feel that the use of the UGS provided them with an opportunity to become aware of the existence of the nature around them (Model 3G). In addition, telecommuters (OR = 1.748, p < 0.001) and older adults (OR = 1.720, p < 0.001) had a significantly better understanding of positive aspects of their neighbourhoods through the use of UGS (Model 3H).

Discussion

Use of UGS during the pandemic

This study revealed that 46% of the respondents used UGS during the first wave of the COVID-19 pandemic in Tokyo. Given that 88% of respondents used them in Brisbane[66], the use of UGS in Tokyo was relatively low. This difference may be due to the fact that the per capita park area in Tokyo is smaller than in Brisbane[67,68], and consequently the habit of using UGS on a daily basis is less popular.

Focusing on the perceptions by users of UGS, the results showed that relatively more people valued stress relief and fewer people valued human connection during the pandemic. This suggests that mental health may have improved

---

[66] Berdejo-Espinola et al., "Urban Green Space Use During a Time of Stress: A Case Study During the COVID-19 Pandemic in Brisbane, Australia."
[67] Bureau of Construction, Tokyo Metropolitan Government, "Parks in Tokyo."
[68] Rupprecht and Byrne, "Informal Urban Green-Space: Comparison of Quantity and Characteristics in Brisbane, Australia and Sapporo, Japan."

through the use of UGS, while social health may have been less likely to improve. These results are in common with the findings of the Brisbane study by Berdejo-Espinola et al.[69]. However, Xie concluded that the users of UGS satisfied their social interaction needs in Chengdu[70]. Berdejo-Espinola et al.[71] explains this difference as being due to the strictness of behavioural restrictions; in Brisbane, the restriction that only one person from the same household could go out is stricter than in Chengdu. Tokyo's behavioural restrictions are not as strict as Brisbane's, but rather similar to Chengdu's[72,73]. Therefore, not only factors related to the COVID-19 pandemic, but also cultural differences in the use of UGS may have influenced the results.

Although the number of users of UGS in Tokyo is small compared to those in other countries, the use of UGS still has a positive effect on the users. Considering the health benefits of UGS, it is worthwhile to open privately owned UGS as well, in case similar restrictions on behaviour are required in the future.

Characteristics of users of UGS during the pandemic

This study reveals who used UGS frequently during the first wave of COVID-19 in Tokyo, Japan. Telecommuters, older adults, and families with children were each significantly correlated with the use of UGS (Model 1A). Telecommuters were significantly correlated with new use of UGS, while older adults and families with children were not significantly correlated (Model 1B). The drastic change in work styles associated with the pandemic may have consequently triggered the use of UGS by telecommuters.

Telecommuters will need to be rethought of as new users of UGS. Several prepandemic studies have discussed the relationship between life stage and the use of UGS[74], and it has been found that age[75,76] and the presence of having

---

[69] Berdejo-Espinola et al., "Urban Green Space Use During a Time of Stress: A Case Study During the COVID-19 Pandemic in Brisbane, Australia."

[70] Xie et al., "Urban Parks as Green Buffers During the COVID-19 Pandemic."

[71] Berdejo-Espinola et al., "Urban Green Space Use During a Time of Stress: A Case Study During the COVID-19 Pandemic in Brisbane, Australia."

[72] Tashiro and Shaw, "COVID-19 Pandemic Response in Japan: What Is Behind the Initial Flattening of the Curve?"

[73] Hale and Webster, "Oxford Covid-19 Government Response Tracker."

[74] Sanesi and Chiarello, "Residents and Urban Green Spaces: The Case of Bari."

[75] Schipperijn et al., "Factors Influencing the Use of Green Space: Results from a Danish National Representative Survey."

[76] Sreetheran, "Exploring the Urban Park Use, Preference and Behaviours Among the Residents of Kuala Lumpur, Malaysia."

children[77, 78, 79] strongly influence the use of UGS. The results of this study for Tokyo during the emergency period also showed that the older adults and families with children frequently used UGS. The relationship between work style and UGS use has only been discussed by Boyd et al.[80], who conducted interviews with individuals regarding their reasons for not using UGS in England, and they found that the most common response was because they were "too busy at work". However, in this study of Tokyo during the emergency period, there was no correlation between decreased time at work and the use of UGS. Independent of the decrease in time spent working, there was a significant correlation between telecommuters and the use of UGS (Model 1A). Even if workers believe that they do not use UGS because they are too busy working, it does not seem likely that they will use UGS if their work hours simply decrease. Whether workers use UGS or not is not only influenced by the time they work but also by their work style.

Telecommuters appear to have a different preference for UGS compared to those who had been frequent users of UGS continuously before the pandemic. For example, there is a significant positive correlation between telecommuters and the use of temple and shrine land, but no significant correlation between older adults and families with children (Model 2E). Meanwhile, older adults and families with children have a significant positive correlation with the use of small parks, but there is no significant correlation among telecommuters (Model 2A). Older adults and families with children significantly felt a connection to others through the use of UGS, but there is no significant correlation for telecommuters (Model 3D). Telecommuters may have avoided small parks crowded and instead used shrines and temples where they could spend time more quietly.

---

[77] Schipperijn et al., "Influences on the Use of Urban Green Space - a Case Study in Odense, Denmark."

[78] Jim and Chen, "Recreation-amenity Use and Contingent Valuation of Urban Greenspaces in Guangzhou, China."

[79] Wong, "Urban Park Visiting Habits and Leisure Activities of Residents in Hong Kong, China."

[80] Boyd et al., "Who Doesn't Visit Natural Environments for Recreation and Why: A Population Representative Analysis of Spatial, Individual and Temporal Factors Among Adults in England."

	Model 3A			Model 3B			Model 3C		
	Felt Satisfied with UGS			Useful for Stress Relief			Reduced Loneliness		
	Odds Ratio	Std. Error	p-Value	Odds Ratio	Std. Error	p-Value	Odds Ratio	Std. Error	p-Value
Intercept	0.912	0.166	0.580	1.366	0.166	0.060	0.374	0.188	0.000***
Telecommuter	1.448	0.133	0.005**	1.259	0.132	0.082	1.219	0.150	0.186
Older adult	1.184	0.147	0.251	1.100	0.146	0.516	1.055	0.173	0.757
Family with children	0.987	0.149	0.928	0.830	0.148	0.210	1.335	0.163	0.077
Male	0.805	0.114	0.057	0.660	0.114	0.000***	0.712	0.129	0.009**
Living with someone	1.379	0.135	0.017*	1.281	0.135	0.067	0.939	0.155	0.684
Dog owner	0.629	0.200	0.021*	0.714	0.200	0.092	0.767	0.249	0.287
Living in suburbs	1.296	0.105	0.014*	0.979	0.105	0.836	0.977	0.121	0.844
Not worker	0.923	0.148	0.588	0.871	0.148	0.353	0.837	0.175	0.307
Decreased worktime	0.956	0.116	0.698	0.973	0.116	0.816	1.102	0.131	0.456
UGS: urban green space. * $p \leq 0.05$; ** $p \leq 0.01$; *** $p \leq 0.001$									

Table 4. Evaluation of use of UGS and user characteristics (Model 3)

	Model 3D			Model 3E			Model 3F		
	Felt a Connection with Others			Distancing Can Be Maintained			Able to Use UGS without Being Self-Conscious		
	Odds Ratio	Std. Error	p-Value	Odds Ratio	Std. Error	p-Value	Odds Ratio	Std. Error	p-Value
Intercept	0.352	0.195	0.000***	1.067	0.169	0.702	0.995	0.168	0.975
Telecommuter	0.940	0.158	0.696	1.008	0.134	0.952	1.153	0.134	0.285
Older adult	1.507	0.175	0.019*	2.020	0.156	0.000***	2.176	0.154	0.000***
Family with children	1.895	0.169	0.000***	1.043	0.149	0.780	0.845	0.148	0.255
Male	0.783	0.135	0.070	0.994	0.116	0.961	1.143	0.114	0.241
Living with someone	0.859	0.162	0.348	1.173	0.137	0.245	0.968	0.137	0.815
Dog owner	0.812	0.258	0.420	1.176	0.210	0.440	1.329	0.209	0.172
Living in suburbs	0.793	0.125	0.064	1.494	0.108	0.000***	1.419	0.107	0.001**
Not worker	0.868	0.177	0.423	0.971	0.154	0.850	0.863	0.152	0.334
Decreased worktime	1.020	0.138	0.886	0.734	0.117	0.008**	0.719	0.116	0.005**
UGS: urban green space. * $p \leq 0.05$; ** $p \leq 0.01$; *** $p \leq 0.001$									

Table 4. Evaluation of use of UGS and user characteristics (Model 3)

	Model 3G			Model 3H		
	Noticed Nature in Close Proximity			Noticed Positive Aspects of my Neighbourhood		
	Odds Ratio	Std. Error	p-Value	Odds Ratio	Std. Error	p-Value
Intercept	0.917	0.169	0.607	0.840	0.168	0.301
Telecommuter	1.506	0.136	0.003**	1.748	0.135	0.000***
Older adult	1.570	0.151	0.003**	1.720	0.149	0.000***
Family with children	1.043	0.151	0.778	1.131	0.149	0.408
Male	0.419	0.117	0.000***	0.470	0.116	0.000***
Living with someone	0.970	0.139	0.825	1.135	0.137	0.355
Dog owner	0.549	0.222	0.007**	0.660	0.209	0.047*
Living in suburbs	1.077	0.108	0.438	0.957	0.106	0.678
Not worker	0.802	0.154	0.152	0.991	0.151	0.952
Decreased worktime	1.162	0.118	0.203	1.144	0.117	0.249
UGS: urban green space. * $p \leq 0.05$; ** $p \leq 0.01$; *** $p \leq 0.001$						

Table 4. Evaluation of use of UGS and user characteristics (Model 3)

Post-COVID-19 planning for UGS

The answer to the question of who uses UGS frequently is not a fixed one determined by life stage, but should be seen as a dynamic one that changes with time and social conditions. Several studies have identified the characteristics of users of UGS[81,82]. However, telecommuters, who are the focus of this study as users of UGS, engage in a new work style made possible by the development of information and communications technology. In addition, the COVID-19 pandemic led many companies to introduce telecommuting systems[83]. Therefore, the use of UGS by telecommuters can be regarded as part of a new-age lifestyle.

If city planners assume that the users of UGS will change due to technological development and social conditions, then future UGS planning should incorporate a perspective of responding to change. Conventional UGS planning in general has aimed to identify the image of the users of UGS and to develop UGS that are comfortable for that target. However, if the user base changes as society changes, as this study shows, the preference for UGS can also change. With this in mind, it would be desirable for city planners to renovate UGS in

---

[81] Kaczynski and Henderson, "Environmental Correlates of Physical Activity: A Review of Evidence About Parks and Recreation."

[82] Kloek et al., "Shifting Workstyle to Teleworking as a New Normal in Face of COVID-19: Analysis with the Model Introducing Intercity Movement and Behavioral Pattern."

[83] Eurofound, "Living, Working and COVID-19 Dataset, Dublin."

response to changes in users in the short term, and in the long term, to aim for a state in which a wide variety of UGS are available to residents so that they can respond to changes in the user base.

In the wake of the pandemic, it is important to design and manage UGS that consider the characteristics of telecommuters. The introduction of telecommuting systems by companies during the COVID-19 pandemic was an effective option to continue business activities while protecting employees from infection risks[84]. However, some studies have shown that telecommuters during the pandemic were at a higher risk of decreased psychological well-being than those who commuted[85]. While telecommuters were more likely to be at risk for health risks, they may have used UGS to improve their health status. The results of this study showed that telecommuters who used UGS tended to feel that their anxiety and stress were alleviated (Model 3B). If telecommuters are considered to have been important supporters of economic activities during the pandemic, it is necessary to discuss how UGS can be effective in reducing their health risks. For example, small parks in neighbourhood are basically designed for children and/or older adults and playground equipment and health devices are installed. However, considering the results of this study, it is worthwhile to take other design options into account, such as planting more trees and creating a quiet atmosphere for stress-relief.

In recent years, there has been an accelerating movement around the world to make a wide variety of open spaces available to citizens. In Japan, for example, a system has been established to encourage companies to renovate parks and to make privately owned vacant land available to citizens[86]. Since it is difficult for governments to purchase land to build parks in urban areas where land prices are high, it is desirable to encourage residents to make a wide variety of UGS available to them by skillfully handling various systems.

Limitations

This was a case study in one Asian megacity, even though it covered both high-density urban centres and low-density suburbs. Therefore, the results are likely to be influenced by the insufficient amount of green space in Tokyo and the cultural

---

[84] Belzunegui-Eraso and Erro-Garcés, "Teleworking in the Context of the Covid-19 Crisis."
[85] Escudero-Castillo, Mato-Díaz and Rodríguez-Álvarez, "Furloughs, Teleworking and Other Work Situations During the COVID-19 Lockdown: Impact on Mental Well-Being."
[86] Ministry of Land, Infrastructure, Transport and Tourism, Government of Japan, "Present Systems and Projects About Parks and Green Spaces."

background of Japanese people's use of UGS. To clarify the characteristics of UGS users in more generic emergencies, comparisons with other cities are important.

The use of internet-based data collection tools can lead to a bias that participants who voluntarily register with the research company are not representative of adults living in Tokyo. However, considering the special circumstances of a pandemic, it was concluded that an online survey was the safest and most reliable method.

This questionnaire survey was conducted in June 2020, immediately after the pandemic was initially announced; this was a time of drastic change in lifestyle, and it will be necessary to determine whether this change is transitory or whether it is something that should be studied for UGS planning in the post-COVID-19 society. Thus, it will be important to compare the results of this study with the results of surveys conducted in the future when more time has passed.

Conclusions

The results of this study contribute to the characterisation of UGS users during the COVID-19 pandemic. An online questionnaire survey of Tokyo residents was conducted to determine whether or not urban residents used UGS, whether or not they used five particular types of UGS, and their evaluation and perception of UGS. A logistic regression analysis was conducted to examine the relationship between the results and the characteristics of the users. The results showed that telecommuters, older adults, and families with children were significantly more likely to use UGS. In addition to the relationship between life stage and UGS use, which has been frequently pointed out in past studies, this study found a correlation between work style and UGS use. This is thought to be a new relationship that was found due to the drastic change in work styles caused by the pandemic. In addition, the preference of telecommuters seems to be different from the preference of older adults and families with children for UGS. Telecommuters do not use small parks significantly as often as older adults and families with children. In addition, telecommuters do not tend to feel connected to other people through the use of UGS as older adults and families with children do. In contrast, telecommuters visit temple and shrine grounds significantly more often, have a higher overall satisfaction with the use of UGS, and appreciate their stress-relieving functions. There were also commonalities such as significantly more frequent use of large parks, greenways, and urban forests. An important finding is that social impacts, such as pandemics, can lead to drastic changes in lifestyle, which in turn can change the users of UGS and their purposes of using UGS.

APPENDIX

Model	Questionnaire	Explanation of the Objective Variable
Model 1 Use of UGS/ Binary variable	Question: "How often did you use UGS during the declaration of the state of emergency?" and "How did the frequency of your use of UGS change during the declaration of the state of emergency compared to before?"	- 1A "user of UGS"; Respondents who use UGS "several times a month," "once or twice a week," "three or four times a week," or "almost every day." - 1B "New user of UGS"; Change in frequency of use of UGS: "No use before, used for the first time/after a long time during the emergency period."
Model 2 Availability of UGS by type of use/Binary variable	Question: "How often did you use the following UGS (small park/ large park/greenway/urban forest/ temple/shrine) during the period when the state of emergency was declared?"	- 2A "Small Park"; Respondents who use a small park/ plaza (with some playground equipment and benches) "several times a month," "once or twice a week," "three or four times a week," or "almost every day." - 2B "Large Park"; Respondents who use large parks and squares (sports facilities and large open spaces of some size) "several times a month," "once or twice a week," "three or four times a week," or "almost every day." - 2C "Greenway"; Respondents who use greenways, riverbeds, and riverside paths "several times a month," "once or twice a week," "three or four times a week," or "almost every day." - 2D "Urban Forest"; Respondents who use woodlands and thickets "several times a month," "once or twice a week," "three or four times a week," or "almost every day." - 2E "Temple and Shrine"; Respondents who use precincts of temples and shrines "several times a month," "once or twice a week," "three or four times a week," or "almost every day."
Model 3 Evaluation and recognition of the use of UGS/Binary variable	Question to be answered only by users of UGS: „During the period of the declaration of a state of emergency, how did you feel when you used UGS?"	- 3A "Felt satisfied with UGS"; Responded "very much agree" or "agree" to the question "I was satisfied with exercising or resting in an urban green space." - 3B "Useful for stress relief"; Responded „very much agree" or "agree" to the question "I felt relieved of anxiety and stress." - 3C "Reduced loneliness"; Responded "very much agree" or "agree" to the question "I felt less lonely." - 3D "Felt a connection with others"; Responded "very much agree" or "agree" to the question "I felt connected to others in a relaxed way." - 3E "Distancing can be maintained"; Responded "very much agree" or "agree" to the question "I was able to maintain a sufficient physical distance in the park green space." - 3F "Able to use UGS without being self-conscious"; Responded "very much agree" or "agree" to the question "I was able to use the UGS without worrying about the eyes around me." - 3G "Noticed nature in close proximity"; Responded "very much agree" or "agree" to the question "It was an opportunity for me to become aware of the existence of nature around me that I had not noticed before." - 3H "Noticed positive aspects of my neighbourhood"; Responded "very much agree" or "agree" to the question "It was an opportunity for me to become aware of the good qualities of the area where I live."

Table A1: Explanation of the study models

Author(s) and Year of Publication	Target and Sample Size	Association(s)
Jim and Chen, 2006	Guangzhou, China; N = 340	older adults, group use, with children
Sanesi and Chiarello, 2006	Bari, Italy; N = 230	suburban residents, 25–44 years old, married
Wong, 2009	Hong Kong, China; N = 758	over 60 years old, married, with children
Schipperijn et al., 2010a	Denmark; N = 21,832	elderly males, more years of education, ethnic Danes
Schipperijn et al., 2010b	Odense, Denmark; N = 1305	with children under 6 years old, dog owners, older adults
Wendel et al., 2012	Santa Cruz, Bolivia; N = 281	male
Sang et al., 2016	Gothenburg, Sweden; N = 1347	female
Sreetheran, 2017	Kuala Lumpur, Malaysia; N = 669	young adults *, group use *
Boyd et al., 2018	England; N = 63,891	male, young, Caucasian, non-full-time worker, married or cohabiting, with children, dog owner

Table A2: Relationship between use of UGS and personal attributes (* no statistical analysis)

Variable	Respondents	Description	Reference(s)
Telecommuter	1152 (37%)	Work style during the emergency period is telecommuting at least one day a week.	
Older Adult	728 (23%)	Age is 65 years or older	Schipperijn et al., 2010a; Schipperijn et al., 2010b; Jim and Chen, 2006; Wong, 2009
Family with Children	434 (14%)	Age between 20 and 45 years old, and living with children	Schipperijn et al., 2010b; Jim and Chen, 2006; Wong, 2009; Boyd et al. 2018
Man	1647 (53%)	The gender is male	Boyd et al., 2018; Wendel et al., 2012
Living with Someone	2329 (75%)	Except for single occupants	Wong, 2009; Boyd et al., 2018; Sanesi and Chiarello, 2006
Dog Owner	188 (6%)	Living with a dog	Schipperijn et al., 2010b
Living in Suburbs	1541 (50%)	Selecting the Tama suburbs as their residence	Sanesi and Chiarello, 2006
Not Worker	1011 (33%)	Not working during the emergency period	Boyd et al., 2018
Decreased worktime	980 (32%)	Slight decrease or decrease in work hours during the emergency period.	

Table A3: Details of the explanatory variables

	Total	
	n	%
Total (all telecommuters)	1132	100%
Telecommuting since before the pandemic	110	10%
Start telecommuting during the pandemic	1022	90%
Telecommuting almost every day	686	61%
Telecommuting up to one day per week	446	39%

Table A4: Telecommuting experience

Bibliography

Agency for Cultural Affairs, Government of Japan. "Religious Statistics Database 2020." Accessed August 3, 2021. https://www.bunka.go.jp/tokei_hakusho_shuppan/tokeichosa/shumu/index.html.

Bedimo-Rung, Ariane L., Andrew J. Mowen, and Deborah A. Cohen. "The Significance of Parks to Physical Activity and Public Health: A Conceptual Model." American journal of preventive medicine 28, 2 Suppl 2 (2005): 159–68. https://doi.org/10.1016/j.amepre.2004.10.024.

Belzunegui-Eraso, Angel, and Amaya Erro-Garcés. "Teleworking in the Context of the Covid-19 Crisis." Sustainability 12, no. 9 (2020): 3662. https://doi.org/10.3390/su12093662.

Berdejo-Espinola, Violeta, Andrés F. Suárez-Castro, Tatsuya Amano, Kelly S. Fielding, Rachel Rui Ying Oh, and Richard A. Fuller. "Urban Green Space Use During a Time of Stress: A Case Study During the COVID-19 Pandemic in Brisbane, Australia." People and nature (Hoboken, N.J.) 3, no. 3 (2021): 597–609. https://doi.org/10.1002/pan3.10218.

Boyd, Francesca, Mathew P. White, Sarah L. Bell, and Jim Burt. "Who Doesn't Visit Natural Environments for Recreation and Why: A Population Representative Analysis of Spatial, Individual and Temporal Factors Among Adults in England." Landscape and Urban Planning 175 (2018): 102–13. https://doi.org/10.1016/j.landurbplan.2018.03.016. https://www.sciencedirect.com/science/article/pii/S0169204618300914.

Bureau of Construction, Tokyo Metropolitan Government. "Urban Green Space Database 2020." Accessed June 30, 2021. https://www.kensetsu.metro.tokyo.lg.jp/content/000049137.pdf.

Bureau of Construction, Tokyo Metropolitan Government. "Parks in Tokyo." Accessed June 30, 2021. https://www.kensetsu.metro.tokyo.lg.jp/english/jigyo/park/01.html.

Cabinet Secretariat, Government of Japan. "About the New Influenza Special Measures Act, COVID-19 Information and Resources." Accessed June 30, 2021. https://corona.go.jp/news/news_20200405_19.html.

Cox, Daniel T. C., Danielle F. Shanahan, Hannah L. Hudson, Kate E. Plummer, Gavin M. Siriwardena, Richard A. Fuller, Karen Anderson, Steven Hancock, and Kevin J. Gaston. "Doses of Neighborhood Nature: The Benefits for Mental Health of Living with Nature." BioScience 67, no. 2 (2017): 147–155. https://doi.org/10.1093/biosci/biw173.

Escudero-Castillo, Israel, Fco. Javier Mato-Díaz, and Ana Rodriguez-Alvarez. "Furloughs, Teleworking and Other Work Situations During the COVID-19 Lockdown: Impact on Mental Well-Being." International Journal of Environmental Research and Public Health 18, no. 6 (2021). https://doi.org/10.3390/ijerph18062898.

Eurofound. "Living, Working and COVID-19 Dataset, Dublin." Accessed June 30, 2021. http://eurofound.link/covid19data.

Geng, Dehui Christina, John Innes, Wanli Wu, and Guangyu Wang. "Impacts of COVID-19 Pandemic on Urban Park Visitation: A Global Analysis." Journal of forestry research 32, no. 2 (2021): 553–67. https://doi.org/10.1007/s11676-020-01249-w.

Grilli, Gianluca, Gretta Mohan, and John Curtis. "Public Park Attributes, Park Visits, and Associated Health Status." Landscape and Urban Planning 199 (2020): 103814. https://doi.org/10.1016/j.landurbplan.2020.103814.

Hale, Thomas, Noam Angrist, Rafael Goldszmidt, Beatriz Kira, Anna Petherick, Toby Phillips, Samuel Webster et al. "A Global Panel Database of Pandemic Policies (Oxford COVID-19 Government Response Tracker)." Accessed July 27, 2021. www.bsg.ox.ac.uk/covidtracker.

Hale, Thomas, and Samuel Webster. "Oxford Covid-19 Government Response Tracker."

Hino, Kimihiro, and Yasushi Asami. "Change in Walking Steps and Association with Built Environments During the COVID-19 State of Emergency: A Longitudinal Comparison with the First Half of 2019 in Yokohama, Japan." Health & Place 69 (2021): 102544. https://doi.org/10.1016/j.healthplace.2021.102544.

Jim, C. Y., and Wendy Y. Chen. "Recreation–amenity Use and Contingent Valuation of Urban Greenspaces in Guangzhou, China." Landscape and Urban Planning 75, no. 1 (2006): 81–96. https://doi.org/10.1016/j.landurbplan.2004.08.008.

Kaczynski, Andrew T., and Karla A. Henderson. "Environmental Correlates of Physical Activity: A Review of Evidence About Parks and Recreation." Leisure Sciences 29, no. 4 (2007): 315–54. https://doi.org/10.1080/01490400701394865.

Karako, Kenji, Peipei Song, Yu Chen, and Wei Tang. "Shifting Workstyle to Teleworking as a New Normal in Face of COVID-19: Analysis with the Model Introducing Intercity Movement and Behavioral Pattern." Annals of translational medicine 8, no. 17 (2020): 1056. https://doi.org/10.21037/atm-20-5334.

Kardan, Omid, Peter Gozdyra, Bratislav Misic, Faisal Moola, Lyle J. Palmer, Tomáš Paus, and Marc G. Berman. "Neighborhood Greenspace and Health in a Large Urban Center." Scientific reports 5 (2015): 11610. https://doi.org/10.1038/srep11610.

Kloek, Marjolein E., Arjen E. Buijs, Jan J. Boersema, and Matthijs G. C. Schouten. "Crossing Borders: Review of Concepts and Approaches in Research on Greenspace, Immigration and Society in Northwest European Countries." Landscape Research 38, no. 1 (2013): 117–40. https://doi.org/10.1080/01426397.2012.690861.

Korpela, K., K. Borodulin, M. Neuvonen, O. Paronen, and L. Tyrväinen. "Analyzing the Mediators Between Nature-Based Outdoor Recreation and Emotional Well-Being." Journal of Environmental Psychology 37 (2014): 1–7. https://doi.org/10.1016/j.jenvp.2013.11.003.

Lafortezza, Raffaele, Giuseppe Carrus, Giovanni Sanesi, and Clive Davies. "Benefits and Well-Being Perceived by People Visiting Green Spaces in Periods of Heat Stress." Urban Forestry & Urban Greening 8, no. 2 (2009): 97–108. https://doi.org/10.1016/j.ufug.2009.02.003. https://www.sciencedirect.com/science/article/pii/S1618866709000168.

Lu, Yi, Jianting Zhao, Xueying Wu, and Siu Ming Lo. "Escaping to Nature During a Pandemic: A Natural Experiment in Asian Cities During the COVID-19 Pandemic with Big Social Media Data." Science of The Total Environment 777 (2021): 146092. https://doi.org/10.1016/j.scitotenv.2021.146092.

Mathieu, Eduard, Hannah Ritchie, Lucas Rodés-Guro, Cameron Appel, Daniel Gavrilov, Charlie Giattino, Joe Hasell et al. "OurWorld in Data." Accessed August 24, 2021. https://ourworldindata.org/coronavirus.

Mayen Huerta, Carolina, and Ariane Utomo. "Evaluating the Association Between Urban Green Spaces and Subjective Well-Being in Mexico City During the COVID-19 Pandemic." Health & Place 70 (2021): 102606. https://doi.org/10.1016/j.healthplace.2021.102606.

Ministry of Land, Infrastructure, Transport and Tourism, Government of Japan. "Present Systems and Projects About Parks and Green Spaces." Accessed June 30, 2021. https://www.mlit.go.jp/common/000996962.pdf.

Ode Sang, Åsa, Igor Knez, Bengt Gunnarsson, and Marcus Hedblom. "The Effects of Naturalness, Gender, and Age on How Urban Green Space Is Perceived and Used." Urban Forestry & Urban Greening 18 (2016): 268–76. https://doi.org/10.1016/j.ufug.2016.06.008.

Organisation for Economic Co-Operation and Development. "Work-Life Balance." http://www.oecdbetterlifeindex.org/topics/work-life-balance.

Peduzzi, Peter, John Concato, Elizabeth Kemper, Theodore R. Holford, and Alvan R. Feinstein. "A Simulation Study of the Number of Events Per Variable in Logistic Regression Analysis." Journal of clinical epidemiology 49, no. 12 (1996): 1373–79. https://doi.org/10.1016/s0895-4356(96)00236-3.

Pérez-Urrestarazu, Luis, Maria P. Kaltsidi, Panayiotis A. Nektarios, Georgios Markakis, Vivian Loges, Katia Perini, and Rafael Fernández-Cañero. "Particularities of Having Plants at Home During the Confinement Due to the COVID-19 Pandemic." Urban Forestry & Urban Greening 59 (2021): 126919. https://doi.org/10.1016/j.ufug.2020.126919.

Poortinga, Wouter, Natasha Bird, Britt Hallingberg, Rhiannon Phillips, and Denitza Williams. "The Role of Perceived Public and Private Green Space in Subjective Health and Wellbeing During and After the First Peak of the COVID-19 Outbreak." Landscape and Urban Planning 211 (2021): 104092. https://doi.org/10.1016/j.landurbplan.2021.104092.

Rupprecht, Christoph D.D., and Jason A. Byrne. "Informal Urban Green-Space: Comparison of Quantity and Characteristics in Brisbane, Australia and Sapporo, Japan." PLoS one 9, no. 6 (2014): e99784. https://doi.org/10.1371/journal.pone.0099784.

Sanesi, Giovanni, and Francesco Chiarello. "Residents and Urban Green Spaces: The Case of Bari." Urban Forestry & Urban Greening 4, no. 3 (2006): 125-34. https://doi.org/10.1016/j.ufug.2005.12.001. https://www.sciencedirect.com/science/article/pii/S1618866705000531.

Schipperijn, Jasper, Ola Ekholm, Ulrika K. Stigsdotter, Mette Toftager, Peter Bentsen, Finn Kamper-Jørgensen, and Thomas B. Randrup. "Factors Influencing the Use of Green Space: Results from a Danish National Representative Survey." Landscape and Urban Planning 95, no. 3 (2010): 130-37. https://doi.org/10.1016/j.landurbplan.2009.12.010. https://www.sciencedirect.com/science/article/pii/S016920460900245X.

Schipperijn, Jasper, Ulrika K. Stigsdotter, Thomas B. Randrup, and Jens Troelsen. "Influences on the Use of Urban Green Space - a Case Study in Odense, Denmark." Urban Forestry & Urban Greening 9, no. 1 (2010): 25-32. https://doi.org/10.1016/j.ufug.2009.09.002.

Shanahan, Danielle F., Robert Bush, Kevin J. Gaston, Brenda B. Lin, Julie Dean, Elizabeth Barber, and Richard A. Fuller. "Health Benefits from Nature Experiences Depend on Dose." Scientific reports 6 (2016): 28551. https://doi.org/10.1038/srep28551.

Soga, Masashi, Maldwyn J. Evans, Kazuaki Tsuchiya, and Yuya Fukano. "A Room with a Green View: The Importance of Nearby Nature for Mental Health During the COVID-19 Pandemic." Ecological applications a publication of the Ecological Society of America 31, no. 2 (2021): e2248. https://doi.org/10.1002/eap.2248.

Sreetheran, Maruthaveeran. "Exploring the Urban Park Use, Preference and Behaviours Among the Residents of Kuala Lumpur, Malaysia." Urban Forestry & Urban Greening 25 (2017): 85-93. https://doi.org/10.1016/j.ufug.2017.05.003. https://www.sciencedirect.com/science/article/pii/S1618866716303193.

Takano, T., K. Nakamura, and M. Watanabe. "Urban Residential Environments and Senior Citizens' Longevity in Megacity Areas: The Importance of Walkable Green Spaces." Journal of epidemiology and community health 56, no. 12 (2002): 913-18. https://doi.org/10.1136/jech.56.12.913.

Tashiro, Ai, and Rajib Shaw. "COVID-19 Pandemic Response in Japan: What Is Behind the Initial Flattening of the Curve?" Sustainability 12, no. 13 (2020): 5250. https://doi.org/10.3390/su12135250.

Tokyo Metropolitan Government. "Message to the People of Tokyo: Refrain from Going Out at Night (Message from the Governor)." Accessed June 24, 2021. https://www.metro.tokyo.lg.jp/english/governor/act/2020/0206_00.html.

Tokyo Metropolitan Government. "Results of the Urgent Survey About Telework Introduction Rate." Accessed June 24, 2021. Results of the Urgent Survey about Telework Introduction Rate.

Ugolini, Francesca, Luciano Massetti, Pedro Calaza-Martínez, Paloma Cariñanos, Cynnamon Dobbs, Silvija Krajter Ostoić, and Ana Marija Marin et al. "Effects of the COVID-19 Pandemic on the Use and Perceptions of Urban Green Space: An International Exploratory Study." Urban Forestry & Urban Greening 56 (2020): 126888. https://doi.org/10.1016/j.ufug.2020.126888.

United Nations, Department of Economic and Social Affairs, Population Division. "World Population Ageing 2019: Highlights (ST/ESA/SER.A/430)." Accessed August 30, 2021. https://www.un.org/en/development/desa/population/publications/pdf/ageing/WorldPopulationAgeing2019-Highlights.pdf.

Venter, Zander S., David N. Barton, Vegard Gundersen, Helene Figari, and Megan Nowell. "Urban Nature in a Time of Crisis: Recreational Use of Green Space Increases During the COVID-19 Outbreak in Oslo, Norway." Environmental Research Letters 15, no. 10 (2020): 104075. https://doi.org/10.1088/1748-9326/abb396.

Verity, Robert, Lucy C. Okell, Ilaria Dorigatti, Peter Winskill, Charles Whittaker, Natsuko Imai, and Gina Cuomo-Dannenburg et al. "Estimates of the Severity of Coronavirus Disease 2019: A Model-Based Analysis." The Lancet. Infectious diseases 20, no. 6 (2020): 669–77. https://doi.org/10.1016/S1473-3099(20)30243-7.

Ward Thompson, Catharine, Jenny Roe, Peter Aspinall, Richard Mitchell, Angela Clow, and David Miller. "More Green Space Is Linked to Less Stress in Deprived Communities: Evidence from Salivary Cortisol Patterns." Landscape and Urban Planning 105, no. 3 (2012): 221–29. https://doi.org/10.1016/j.landurbplan.2011.12.015.

Wong, Koon Kwai. "Urban Park Visiting Habits and Leisure Activities of Residents in Hong Kong, China." Managing Leisure 14, no. 2 (2009): 125–40. https://doi.org/10.1080/13606710902752653.

World Health Organization. "Statement on the Second Meeting of the International Health Regulations (2005) Emergency Committee Regarding the Outbreak of Novel Coronavirus (2019-NCoV)." Accessed June 24, 2021. https://www.who.int/news/item/30-01-2020-statement-on-the-second-meeting-of-the-international-health-regulations-(2005)-emergency-committeeregarding-the-outbreak-of-novel-coronavirus-(2019-ncov).

Wright Wendel, Heather E., Rebecca K. Zarger, and James R. Mihelcic. "Accessibility and Usability: Green Space Preferences, Perceptions, and Barriers in a Rapidly Urbanizing City in Latin America." Landscape and Urban Planning 107, no. 3 (2012): 272–82. https://doi.org/10.1016/j.landurbplan.2012.06.003.

Xie, Jing, Shixian Luo, Katsunori Furuya, and Dajiang Sun. "Urban Parks as Green Buffers During the COVID-19 Pandemic." Sustainability 12, no. 17 (2020): 6751. https://doi.org/10.3390/su12176751.

The Contributors

Noriko AKITA is a Professor at the Department of Environmental Science and Landscape Architecture, Graduate School of Horticulture, Chiba University. Her academic interests include landscape management, urban planning, and land use management. Akita's professional career includes Research Fellow at The University of Tokyo (2004-2008), Associate Professor at Chiba University (2008-2022), and Invited Researcher at CNRS (France) (2022-2023). Her career as a technical advisor includes Member of the Council for Social Infrastructure Development, Ministry of Land, Infrastructure, Transport and Tourism, Fukushima 3.11 Memorial Park Design Review Committee. She has served as an expert in the Diet during the passage process of Japan's watershed flood control laws and was honored by the Minister of Reconstruction in 2018 for her progressive reconstruction efforts following the Great East Japan Earthquake. She was a board member of the Japanese Institute of Landscape Architecture (2018-2021) and currently serves as the board member of the City Planning Institute of Japan (2021-).

Marco AMATI is an Environmental Scientist with a PhD in Planning from the University of Tsukuba (Japan). He is the author of *The City and the Super-organism* (Palgrave, 2021) and has edited three books: *Urban green belts in the 21st Century* (2008); *Exhibitions and the Development of Modern Planning Culture* (2014) with Robert Freestone, and *Conflict and Change in Australia's Peri-Urban Landscapes* (2016) with Andrew Butt and Melissa Kennedy. He works at RMIT University where he teaches Planning History and researches urban forests.

Irene BITTNER was between 2009 and 2020 Researcher and Lecturer at the University of Vienna, at the University of Natural Resources and Life Sciences, Vienna, and the University of Graz. Educated as a Landscape Planner she focussed on urban research topics connecting physical activity and active mobility, health, green infrastructure and public space with social aspects. She wrote her doctorate at the University of Natural Resources and Life Sciences, Vienna on *Open space for physical activity, sport and game of adolescents in the compact city* (2018). Between 2020 and 2022 she coordinated the publication series of VCÖ – a public-benefit organisation on sustainable mobility and transport – on topics such as "Climate Factor Travel" (2020), "More Space for Active Mobility" (2021) and "Healthy Cities through healthy mobility"

(2022). She now works as an expert at the Austrian Energy Agency within the federal climate initiative "klimaaktiv mobil" to put sustainable mobility into practice.

Meinhard BREILING studied landscape architecture at BOKU Wien (Austrian University of Life Sciences, Vienna) where he received his M.Sc. (1988) and PhD (1993). Since 2000 he has worked at the TU Wien (Vienna University of Technology) lecturing on landscape and regional planning at the Faculty of Architecture and Planning and co-ordinating the interfaculty co-operation centre Technology.Tourism. Landscape TTL of TU Wien established in 2005. He has a broad international network and has worked at universities or research centres in Europe (IIASA Laxenburg, BOKU Wien, SLU Alnarp, NMBU Aas, Mendel University Lednice) and Asia (University of Tokyo, Kyoto University, Keio University, University of Hyogo – ALPHA, and Gyeongsang National University, Jinju).

Fabian DEMBSKI is a Research Professor at TalTech (Tallinn University of Technology) and a researcher at HLRS (High-Performance Computing Center Stuttgart). In his research he focuses on topics related inter alia to digital transformation in urban planning, collaborative and participatory decision making processes, spatial analytics, urban simulation and visualisation. Dembski holds a Master's degree in Architecture and a PhD in Spatial Planning from TU Wien and has published on research topics including Global Systems Science, post-oil scenarios, urban digital twins and sustainable transformation strategies. These include, amongst others, a book chapter on digital tools in stakeholder participation for the German energy transition (2020) and a paper on urban digital twins for smart cities and citizens (2020).

Kimihiro HINO is an Associate Professor at the Department of Urban Engineering, The University of Tokyo. His academic interests include healthy urban planning, walkable design, and crime prevention through environmental design (CPTED). Hino's professional career includes: Senior Research Engineer at the Building Research Institute in Japan, Associate Professor of the Cooperative Graduate School of Tsukuba University and Visiting Scholar at the University of Cambridge. In 2021 he published "Active Urban Planning & Design Guide" as the PI of a JSPS-funded research project.

U HIROI is a Professor at The University of Tokyo, and a Visiting Professor at both Nagoya University and Shizuoka University. His academic interests include urban planning and disaster risk reduction. Hiroi's professional career includes: Assistant Professor at The University of Tokyo (2007 to 2012), Associate Professor at the Disaster Mitigation Research Center, Nagoya University (2012 to 2016) and Associate Professor at The University of Tokyo (2016 to 2021). His career as a technical advisor includes being a member of the editorial board of Urban and Regional Planning Review and being vice editor in chief of the Journal of Disaster Information Studies for Japan Society for Disaster Information Studies

The Contributors

Akiko IIDA is a Senior Researcher at the Department of Urban Engineering, The University of Tokyo. She holds a Master's degree in Media and Governance from Keio University and a PhD. in Engineering from The University of Tokyo. Her academic interests include landscape planning, urban ecology, urban food system, green infrastructure, and climate change mitigation and adaptation. She recently published a paper about the contribution of urban agriculture to health and food system resilience during the COVID-19 pandemic (2023 in npj Urban Sustainability). As an urbanist, she also works with local governments and communities on various urban planning and design projects.

Hideki KOIZUMI is a Professor at the Department of Urban Engineering, The University of Tokyo. He also directs the Co-creative Living Lab at the Research Center for Advanced Science and Technology, The University of Tokyo. Koizumi is an expert in collaborative planning, sustainable city planning, and the digital smart city. Koizumi's professional career includes: Assistant Professor at the Science University of Tokyo, Associate Professor at the University of Tokyo, Visiting Scholar at the University of Washington. His career as a Technical Advisor includes: being a member of the Social Infrastructure Development Council of the Ministry of Land, Infrastructure, Transport and Tourism, of the Board for Promoting Future Environmental Cities and of the Digital Agency's Well-being Index Expert Council. Koizumi currently serves as the Head of the Master course in Sustainable Urban Regeneration at The University of Tokyo.

Masayasu KOMIYA is a Professor of Cultural History of Europe, Music Sociology and Comparative Cultural Theory at YNU (Yokohama National University). Furthermore, he organises and comments on classical concert television and radio programmes, including the Vienna Philharmonic's "New Year's Concert", NHK (Nippon Hōsō Kyōkai, Japan Broadcasting Corporation). His publications include: Translation and Compilation of *The Present State of Music in Germany, the Netherlands, and United Provinces by Charles Burney* (Shunju Sha, 2020), *Constanze Mozart, truthfulness and falsehood in the legend of a 'bad wife'* (Kodansha, 2017), *Important but unknown, the shadow existences of music history* (Shunhu Sha, 2013) and *The 'creator' of Mozart: Koechel and Vienna in the 19th century* (Kodan Sha, 2011).

Iris MACH is a Senior Scientist and Head of the Japan Austria Science Exchange Center (JASEC) at TU Wien, which supports and coordinates the scientific exchange of TU Wien with 15 Japanese partner institutions. She completed her Master's degree at TU Wien and prepared her doctoral thesis at the University of Tokyo, supported by a MEXT scholarship of the Japanese Ministry of Education from 2007–2009. Her research interests range from traditional and contemporary Japanese architecture to earthquake-proof buildings and disaster mitigation with publications such as *Traditionelles Wissen und moderne Technologie. Erdbebensicheres Bauen in Japan* (*Traditional knowledge and modern technology. Earthquake-resistant construction in Japan*, Steeldoc,

2011) or *Japan's Architectural Genome. Destruction as a Chance for Renewal* (Int|AR, 2014). In 2017 she received the JSPS Alumni Club Award (JACA) for the promotion of scientific exchange between Japan and the German-speaking area.

Rinpei MIURA is an Associate Professor at the Institute of Urban and Innovation, YNU (Yokohama National University). He holds a PhD in Sociology from the University of Tokyo. His research focuses on urban sociology and regional sociology. He is interested in empirically examining and theorising about the outcomes of social inclusion activities, such as community building and outreach for post-disaster reconstruction, and exploring the challenges involved. Rinpei Miura is the author of the article *Rethinking Gentrification and the Right to the City: The Process and Effect of the Urban Social Movement against Redevelopment in Tokyo* (International Journal of Japanese Sociology 30 (1), 2021).

Akito MURAYAMA is an Associate Professor and the Head of Urban Land Use Planning Unit at Department of Urban Engineering, School of Engineering, The University of Tokyo. He holds a Master's degree and PhD in Urban Engineering from The University of Tokyo. Murayama's research focuses on climate change mitigation and adaptation planning methodology, as well as a framework for district, urban and regional planning. Co-authored books in English include *Living Cities in Japan: Citizens' Movements, Machizukuri and Local Environments* (Routledge, 2007), *Innovations in Collaborative Urban* Regeneration (Springer, 2009), *Urban Resilience – A Transformative Approach* (Springer, 2016), *Towards the Implementation of the New Urban Agenda: Contributions from Japan and Germany to Make Cities More Environmentally Sustainable* (Springer, 2018) and *Urban Systems Design: Creating Sustainable Smart Cities in the Internet of Things Era* (Elsevier, 2020).

Barbara RIEF VERNAY is a Senior Lecturer at TU Wien (Vienna University of Technology). She holds a Master's degree in architecture from TU Wien and a PhD in Urban Geography from Université Paris Ouest Nanterre La Défense/France. Rief Vernay worked for a decade as an architect in different Austrian architectural firms mainly in the field of urban renewal, before she came to urban research. Her scientific work focuses on the development of Central European and European post-socialist cities. She has published papers on the topics of urban politics, urban decay, heritage policies, urban redevelopment strategies, post-fordist culture-led policies and urban history. Rief Vernay is particularly interested in comparative metropolitan research and is co-editor of the book *Wien- Budapest. Stadträume des 20. Jahrhunderts im Vergleich* (*Vienna-Budapest. 20*th *century urban spaces in comparison,* Praesens, 2020).

Keisuke SAKAMOTO is an Assistant Professor at The University of Tokyo. He holds a Master's degree and a PhD of Engineering from The University of Tokyo. His research focuses on inquiry into sustainable urban forms in Tokyo metropolitan areas and Japanese regional cities facing population decline. He has published scientific papers on the topics of urban shrinking phenomena and redevelopment strategies in Japanese cities. An example of his major works is about the patterns of population turnovers in a Japanese regional city (2018, in *Cities*), and his recent work was published on SSRN in 2023, regarding relationships between feasible compact urban forms and land price structures of Japanese regional cities. He also holds a post at the Center for Real Estate Innovation of The University of Tokyo, being particularly interested in socio-spatial analyses using real estate data.

Takeru SHIBAYAMA is a Senior Scientist at the Institute of Transportation, TU Wien (Vienna University of Technology). He studied Civil Engineering with a focus on policy and planning at the University of Tokyo for his Bachelor and Master's degrees, and he holds a PhD in Transport Planning from TU Wien. His research focuses on public transport technologies (planning and policy) with a particular emphasis on sustainable and strategic transport policy. At the beginning of the pandemic, he initiated an international questionnaire survey on the changes of travel behaviour in response to COVID-19 in 21 languages, collecting more than 12,000 responses from over 100 countries. The results were published as the journal paper *Impact of COVID-19 lockdown on commuting: a multi-country perspective* (2021). He is also a co-editor of the book *International Perspectives on Public Transport Responses to COVID-19*, which is expected to be published in 2023.

Toru TERADA is an Associate Professor and the Head of the Landscape and Urban Planning lab. at the Graduate School of Frontier Sciences, The University of Tokyo. He received a Master's degree in Policy and Planning Sciences from the University of Tsukuba in 2008 and a PhD in Environmental Studies from The University of Tokyo in 2011. His field of expertise is policy and planning science in urban and peri-urban areas, considering parks, trees, forests, farmlands, and other green and open spaces as essential to urban landscapes. He and his lab members have recently published scientific papers about biomass production of satoyama woodlands (2020 in Sustainability Sciences), distribution supporting systems in urban agriculture by not-for-profit organisations (2022 in Journal of the City Planning Institute of Japan), and urban tree's ecosystem services and its perception by residents (2023 in Landscape Research Japan Online).

Takahiro YAMAZAKI is a Project Lecturer at the Organisation for Interdisciplinary Research Project, The University of Tokyo. His academic interests include urban planning, landscape planning and landscape ecology. Yamazaki's professional career includes a JSPS Research Fellowship for Young Scientists at Hokkaido University (2015 to 2017), a JSPS Research Fellowship for Young Scientists at The University of Tokyo (2017 to 2019), Visiting Researcher at the Politecnico di Torino, Italy (2018), Project Assistant Professor at The University of Tokyo (2019 to 2021) and Assistant Professor at Kobe Design University (2021 to 2023). His career as a Technical Advisor includes the editorial board of the Architectural Institute of Japan and the selection committee for Kobe community-proposed activities.

Makoto YOKOHARI is a Professor at the Department of Urban Engineering and the Graduate Program in Sustainability Science (GPSS), The University of Tokyo. His academic interests include urban planning, landscape planning and landscape ecology. Yokohari's professional career includes Research Fellow at the National Institute of Agro-Environmental Sciences (1986 to 1998), Visiting Scholar at the University of Guelph, Canada (1992 to 1993), Associate Professor at the University of Tsukuba (1998 to 2004), Professor at the University of Tsukuba (2004 to 2006) and Visiting Scholar at the University of Copenhagen (2015). His career as a technical advisor includes National Capital Region Planning Committee, EXPO2005 Planning Committee, 2020 Tokyo Olympic Games Planning Committee, and the Chair of Agriculture, Forestry and Fisheries Planning Committee of Tokyo Metropolitan Government. Yokohari was the President of the City Planning Institute of Japan (2016 to 2018) and the President of the Japanese Institute of Landscape Architecture (2017 to 2019), and currently serves as the head of the Campus Planning Committee of the University of Tokyo.

HABITAT – INTERNATIONAL
Schriften zur internationalen Stadtentwicklung
hrsg. von Prof. Dr. Peter Herrle, Prof. Dr. Astrid Ley, Dr. Sonja Nebel, Dr. Josefine Fokdal

Marielly Casanova
Social Strategies Building the City
A Re-conceptualization of Social Housing in Latin America
Social housing is a complex system integrated by social, economic, political and city making processes. Social practices in the called social production of the habitat provide clues to understand an alternative way to approach housing solutions in which several dimensions coexist. Through the rationalization of social (self-management), economic (social economy) and urban principles, it was possible the construction of typologies to document and evaluate 3 case studies in Latin America. This book provides a foundation for future research and conception of social housing policies and programs.
vol. 24, 2019, 332 pp., 49,90 €, pb., ISBN-CH 978-3-643-80284-2

Agnes Katharina Müller
Coworking Spaces
Urbane Räume im Kontext flexibler Arbeitswelten
Am Beispiel von Berliner „Coworking Spaces" untersucht Agnes Müller die Raumwirksamkeit einer mobilen und flexiblen Arbeitsgesellschaft. Die Zusammenhänge des besonderen Bürokonzeptes mit einer sich ändernden Arbeitswelt, dem städtischen Raum und seinen kreativen Milieus, sowie Migration und Multilokalität erläutert sie auf drei Maßstabsebenen. Hierin zeigt sich, dass es sich bei diesen Büros um ein „glokales", heterogenes und schnelllebiges Phänomen handelt. Während sich die Büros zunehmend spezialisieren oder auch professionalisieren, nehmen sie Einfluss auf das Stadtleben und die Stadtentwicklung.
Bd. 23, 2018, 298 S., 34,90 €, br., ISBN 978-3-643-14108-8

Shahd Wari
Palestinian Berlin
Perception and Use of Public Space
How do Palestinian immigrants perceive and use the public space in the city of Berlin? Is their perception and use of space homogenous as a group? What are the main patterns of their socio-spatial practices in public spaces? How do they influence the urban landscape of the neighborhoods in which they live? Which factors play a role in their perception and use of public space and how do the hybrid identities of the second and third generations affect their socio-spatial behavior in comparison to the first generation? This book aims to present a study about Palestinian immigrants in Berlin and answer these questions and more about Palestinian identity, socio-spatial practices and use of public space.
vol. 22, 2017, 310 pp., 44,90 €, pb., ISBN-CH 978-3-643-90819-3

Sonja Nebel; Aurel von Richthofen (Eds.)
Urban Oman
Trends and Perspectives of Urbanisation in Muscat Capital Area
The book traces urbanisation patterns in Oman looking at the coastal strip of Muscat Capital Area. This metropolitan region emerged within the last 50 years almost out of nowhere and is now home of the majority of the national and expatriate population of Oman.

LIT Verlag Berlin – Münster – Wien – Zürich – London
Auslieferung Deutschland / Österreich / Schweiz: siehe Impressumsseite

Urbanisation, and the socio-political, economic and environmental aspects attached to it, become an index of the radical spatial transformation of the Sultanate. This process, if managed well, also holds the key to sustainable urban development. Urban Oman invites geographers, planners, urban designers, architects, decision-makers and scholars of Gulf Studies to rethink the emergence of Muscat Capital Area and to embrace the urban Oman.
vol. 21, 2016, 276 pp., 34,90 €, pb., ISBN-CH 3-643-90714-1

Peter Herrle; Josefine Fokdal; Detlev Ipsen (†) (eds.)
Beyond Urbanism
Urban(izing) Villages and the Mega-urban Landscape in the Pearl River Delta in China
Large urban agglomerations have emerged over the past decades and, in some cases, entire rural regions were urbanized in less than a decade. These trends not only reflect an unprecedented quantitative dimension of urbanization but also the emergence of new urban forms – beyond urbanism – thus posing new challenges to regional planners, politicians and urban governance actors.
vol. 20, 2014, 192 pp., 29,90 €, pb., ISBN-CH 978-3-643-90552-9

Beate Ginzel
Bridge the Gap!
Modes of action and cooperation of transnational networks of local communities and their influence on the urban development in the Global South
In the course of a changed understanding of urban management and development cooperation, interest is increasingly being focused on networks. These are more and more recognised as appropriate modes of action and cooperation for the development of multidimensional and flexible actor systems. The author identifies four modes of action and cooperation of transnational networks of local communities by taking the Tanzania Urban Poor Federation (TUPF) as an example. The results provide guidance for the development of network structures bridging existing gaps in the field of urban governance in the Global North and South.
vol. 19, 2015, 336 pp., 39,90 €, pb., ISBN-CH 978-3-643-90533-8

André Alexander
The Traditional Lhasa House
Typology of an Endangered Species
vol. 18, 2013, 416 pp., 69,90 €, pb., ISBN-CH 978-3-643-90203-0

Bettina Bauerfeind; Josefine Fokdal (Eds.)
Bridging Urbanities
Reflections on Urban Design in Shanghai and Berlin
vol. 17, 2011, 160 pp., 24,90 €, pb., ISBN-CH 978-3-643-90131-6

Paola Alfaro d'Alençon; Walter Alejandro Imilan; Lina María Sánchez (Hrsg.)
Lateinamerikanische Städte im Wandel
Zwischen lokaler Stadtgesellschaft und globalem Einfluss
Bd. 16, 2011, 248 S., 29,90 €, br., ISBN 978-3-643-11084-8

Walter Alejandro Imilan
Warriache – Urban Indigenous
Mapuche Migration and Ethnicity in Santiago de Chile
vol. 15, 2011, 280 pp., 24,90 €, pb., ISBN 978-3-643-10475-5

LIT Verlag Berlin – Münster – Wien – Zürich – London
Auslieferung Deutschland / Österreich / Schweiz: siehe Impressumsseite